NATURES (HOME) REMEDY TOOLBOX

JUST ASK.

WHAT THINGS CAN BE FOUND ON
MOST GROCERY SHELVES.

Coach Ez

Table of Contents

A balanced diet that includes a variety of foods, especially those rich in healthy fats and antioxidants, can help you meet your vitamin E requirements. Keep in mind that vitamin E is sensitive to heat and oxygen, so minimizing processing and storage time of foods can help retain their vitamin E content. If you have specific dietary concerns or conditions that affect your vitamin E intake or

Natures (Home) Remedy Toolbox

JUST ASK THINGS CAN BE FOUND ON MOST GROCERY SHELVES.

Healthiest options for ailments, illness, and overall daily health

"

INTRODUCTION:

In a world where modern medicine has made remarkable advancements, it is easy to overlook the incredible healing power that nature has to offer. From ancient civilizations to contemporary holistic practices, humanity has relied on the bountiful gifts of the natural world to soothe ailments, rejuvenate the body, and enhance overall well-being. Welcome to "Nature's Healing Toolbox: A Guide to Natural Remedies."

In this book, we embark on a journey through the rich tapestry of natural remedies that have been cherished by cultures across the globe for centuries. From herbal tinctures to age-old rituals, the wisdom of nature is waiting to be explored and harnessed for your benefit.

Modern life, with its conveniences and technologies, has brought undeniable advantages, but it has also introduced new challenges to our health and well-being. Stress, pollution, and the overuse of synthetic pharmaceuticals have led many to seek alternative paths to wellness. The quest for a comprehensive approach to healing, one that aligns with the rhythms of nature, has never been more relevant.

Coach Ez

is your comprehensive guide to tapping into the vast reservoir of natural remedies. Whether you are interested in relieving everyday ailments, enhancing your immune system, or achieving a greater sense of balance, this book offers a treasure trove of knowledge to aid you on your journey.

Within these pages, you will discover:

1. Introduction

- Explanation of home remedies
- Safety precautions and when to seek professional medical advice.

2. Common Ailments

- Headaches
- Coughs and sore throats
- Fever
- Allergies
- Insomnia

3. Skin and Hair Care

- Acne treatment
- Dry skin remedies
- Dandruff solutions
- Natural hair care

4. Digestive Health

- Remedies for indigestion
- Constipation relief
- Nausea and vomiting
- Heartburn

5. Immune System Boosters

- Homemade herbal teas
- Immune-boosting foods
- Homeopathic remedies

6. First Aid

- Wound care and disinfection
- Bee stings and insect bites
- Burns and minor injuries.

7. Natural Pain Relief

- Back pain remedies
- Toothache relief

1. pharmaceutical drugs. These methods are often less invasive and can have fewer side effects. Here are **some common natural pain relief techniques and Natural pain relief methods can be effective for** managing several types of pain without relying on remedies:

- **Heat:** Applying a warm compress or heating pad can help relax muscles and alleviate pain, especially for muscle aches and joint pain.
- **Cold:** Applying ice packs or cold compresses can reduce inflammation and numb the area, supplying relief for acute injuries or swollen joints.

2. *EXERCISE AND PHYSICAL THERAPY:*

- Regular exercise can help maintain joint flexibility and strengthen muscles, which can reduce pain in conditions like arthritis or lower back pain.
- Physical therapy exercises prescribed by a healthcare professional can target specific areas of pain and improve mobility.

3. Massage Therapy:

PROFESSIONAL MASSAGES OR SELF-MASSAGE TECHNIQUES CAN HELP RELAX TENSE MUSCLES AND PROMOTE BLOOD CIRCULATION, REDUCING PAIN AND STIFFNESS.

4. *ACUPUNCTURE:*

- This traditional Chinese medicine practice involves inserting thin needles into specific points on the body to stimulate energy flow and relieve pain. It is often used for chronic pain conditions.

5. *HERBAL REMEDIES:*

- Certain herbs and botanicals have natural pain-relieving properties. Examples include:

- **Turmeric:** Contains curcumin, which has anti- inflammatory properties.
- **Ginger:** Known for its anti-inflammatory and analgesic effects.
- **Willow Bark:** Contains sailfin, a natural pain reliever similar to aspirin.

6. *AROMATHERAPY:*

- Essential oils like lavender, peppermint, and eucalyptus can be used in aromatherapy to promote relaxation and reduce pain when applied topically or diffused.

7. *MIND-BODY TECHNIQUES:*

- Practices like yoga, tai chi, and meditation can help reduce pain perception by promoting relaxation, improving posture, and increasing body awareness.

8. *DIETARY CHANGES:*

- Anti-inflammatory diets, such as the Mediterranean diet, emphasize foods like fish, fruits, vegetables, and whole grains, which may help reduce pain associated with inflammation.

9. *EPSOM SALT BATHS:*

- Soaking in a warm bath with Epsom salt can relax muscles, ease tension, and provide relief for soreness and muscle pain.

10. CBD and Cannabis: - Cannabidiol (CBD) products derived from hemp or cannabis are gaining popularity for their potential pain-relieving properties. They may help reduce chronic pain and inflammation.

11. Breathing and Relaxation Techniques: - Deep breathing exercises and relaxation techniques can help alleviate stress-related pain and muscle tension.

12. Guided Imagery: - Guided imagery involves visualizing calming and soothing scenes, which can help divert attention away from pain and reduce its perception.

It is important to note that individual responses to natural pain relief methods can vary, and what works for one person may not work as effectively for another. Additionally, consult with a healthcare provider before starting any new pain management regimen, especially if you have chronic or severe pain, to ensure it is safe and appropriate for your specific condition.

Tell me more about herbal remedies.

Herbal remedies involve the use of plants, herbs, and botanical substances for therapeutic purposes. These remedies have been used for centuries in various traditional medicine systems worldwide. Here are some common herbal remedies and their uses:

1. Aloe Vera:

- **Uses:** Aloe vera gel, extracted from the leaves of the aloe plant, is well-known for its soothing properties and is often used topically to

- relieve skin irritations, burns, and minor wounds.

2. Chamomile:

- **Uses:** Chamomile tea or chamomile extracts are used for their calming and anti-inflammatory properties. It is commonly used to alleviate digestive discomfort, promote relaxation, and soothe skin conditions.

3. Echinacea:

- **Uses:** Echinacea is believed to stimulate the immune system and is often used as a natural remedy for colds and respiratory infections. It may also help reduce the severity and duration of symptoms.

4. Ginger:

- **Uses:** Ginger has anti-inflammatory and anti-nausea properties. It is often used to alleviate nausea, motion sickness, and digestive issues, including indigestion and gas.

5. Peppermint:

- **Uses:** Peppermint is known for its ability to relieve digestive discomfort, including indigestion and irritable bowel syndrome (IBS). Peppermint oil can also be applied topically for headaches and muscle pain.

6. Valerian Root:

- **Uses:** Valerian root is used as a natural remedy for anxiety, insomnia, and stress. It may help promote relaxation and improve sleep quality.

7. Turmeric:

- **Uses:** Turmeric contains curcumin, a potent anti-inflammatory compound. It is used to reduce inflammation, alleviate joint pain, and support overall joint health.

8. Ginseng:

- **Uses:** Ginseng is believed to boost energy, improve mental clarity, and enhance physical stamina. It is often used as an adaptogen to combat stress.

9. St. John's Wort:

- **Uses:** St. John's Wort is used as a natural remedy for mild to moderate depression and anxiety. It may help improve mood and reduce symptoms.

10. Saw Palmetto: - Uses: Saw palmetto is commonly used to support prostate health and relieve urinary symptoms associated with benign prostatic hyperplasia (BPH).

11. Milk Thistle: - Uses: Milk thistle is known for its liver-protective properties. It is used to support liver health and detoxification processes.

12. Garlic: - Uses: Garlic is known for its immune-boosting and cardiovascular benefits. It may help reduce blood pressure, lower cholesterol levels, and support overall heart health.

13. Ginkgo Biloba: - Uses: Ginkgo biloba is used to improve cognitive function, enhance memory, and support circulation. It is often recommended for conditions like Alzheimer's disease and age-related cognitive decline.

14. Arnica: - Uses: Arnica is used topically in the form of creams and ointments to relieve muscle pain, bruises, and inflammation.

Coach Ez

It is essential to exercise caution when using herbal remedies, as they can interact with medications or have side effects, especially if not used correctly. If you are considering herbal remedies for a specific health concern, consult with a healthcare professional or a qualified herbalist to ensure their safety and effectiveness for your individual circumstances. Additionally, consider the quality and purity of herbal products, as standardized extracts or reputable brands are often recommended for consistent results.

What are some natural remedies for anxiety?

Natural remedies for anxiety can be effective for managing mild to moderate symptoms of anxiety. However, it is important to note that severe or persistent anxiety should be discussed with a healthcare professional for proper evaluation and treatment. Here are some natural remedies that may help alleviate anxiety:

1. *DEEP BREATHING AND RELAXATION TECHNIQUES:*

   - Practice deep breathing exercises, such as diaphragmatic breathing or the 4-7-8 technique, to calm your nervous system and reduce anxiety.

2. *EXERCISE REGULARLY:*

   - Physical activity releases endorphins, which are natura mood lifters. Aim for at least 30 minutes of moderate exercise most days of the week.

MEDITATION AND MINDFULNESS:

- Meditation and mindfulness practices can help you stay present, reduce rumination, and lower overall stress levels.

3. *YOGA:*

- Yoga combines physical postures, breathing exercises, and meditation to promote relaxation and reduce anxiety.

4. *HERBAL SUPPLEMENTS:*

- Certain herbal supplements like valerian root, passionflower, and kava have calming properties and may help reduce anxiety symptoms. Consult with a healthcare professional before using herbal supplements, especially if you are taking medications.

5. *AROMATHERAPY:*

- Essential oils like lavender, chamomile, and bergamot can be used in aromatherapy to promote relaxation and reduce anxiety. You can diffuse these oils or dilute them and apply them topically.

6. *DIETARY ADJUSTMENTS:*

- Avoid excessive caffeine, sugar, and alcohol, as they can worsen anxiety. A balanced diet rich in whole foods, fruits, vegetables, and lean proteins can support overall mental well-being.

7. *LIMIT STIMULANTS:*

- Reduce or cut stimulants like nicotine and recreational drugs, as they can increase anxiety and panic symptoms.

8. *HERBAL TEAS:*

- Herbal teas like chamomile, lemon balm, and passionflower are known for their calming effects and can be soothing when consumed.

9. *SUPPLEMENTS:*

- Some individuals find relief from anxiety symptoms by taking supplements like magnesium, omega-3 fatty acids, or vitamin B complex. Consult with a healthcare provider before adding supplements to your routine.

10. *LIMIT TECHNOLOGY AND SCREEN TIME:*

- Excessive screen time, especially before bedtime, can contribute to anxiety and disrupted sleep patterns. Consider setting limits on device usage.

11. *JOURNALING:*

- Keeping a journal to express your thoughts and feelings can help you gain insight into your anxiety triggers and find healthy ways to cope.

12. *SLEEP HYGIENE:*

- Prioritize good sleep habits, including a consistent sleep schedule, a comfortable sleep environment, and avoiding caffeine and screens before bedtime.

13. *SOCIAL SUPPORT:*

- Stay connected with friends and family, as social support can be a significant buffer against anxiety. Talking about your feelings and concerns can supply relief.

14. PROFESSIONAL HELP:

- If your anxiety is severe or persistent, or if it significantly changes your daily life, consider seeking help from a mental health professional. Therapy (such as cognitive- behavioral therapy) and, in some cases, medication may be recommended.

Remember that natural remedies for anxiety can be part of a comprehensive self-care plan, but it is essential to tailor your approach to your specific needs and consult with a healthcare provider for guidance, especially if you have any underlying health conditions or concerns.

TELL ME MORE ABOUT MINDFULNESS TECHNIQUES.

Mindfulness techniques are practices that involve paying deliberate and non-judgmental attention to the present moment. These techniques can help reduce stress, improve mental well-being, and enhance overall quality of life. Here are some mindfulness techniques and exercises:

1. *MINDFUL BREATHING:*

- Find a quiet space to sit or lie down comfortably.

- Close your eyes and take a few deep, intentional breaths.

- Pay attention to your breath as it flows in and out of your body.

- Notice the sensation of the breath in your nostrils, the rise and fall of your chest or abdomen, and the rhythm of your breath.

- When your mind wanders (as it inevitably will), gently bring your focus back to your breath without judgment.

2. *BODY SCAN MEDITATION:*

- Lie down or sit in a comfortable position.

- Start at the top of your head and slowly move your attention down through your body.

- Pay attention to any sensations, tension, or discomfort in each body part as you progress.

- Relax and release tension as you become aware of it.

3. *MINDFUL EATING:*

- Choose a small piece of food, such as a raisin or a piece of fruit.

- Examine the food using all your senses. Notice its texture, color, smell, and any sounds it makes.

- Take a small bite and savor the taste, texture, and flavors without rushing.

- Pay attention to how your body responds to each bite.

4. WALKING MEDITATION:

- Go for a walk at a slow and deliberate pace, either indoors or outdoors.
- Focus on the sensation of each step as your foot lifts, moves, and touches the ground.
- Pay attention to your breath as you walk.
- If your mind wanders, gently bring your focus back to the sensations of walking and breathing.

5. MINDFUL OBSERVATION:

- Choose an object in your environment, such as a flower, a tree, or a piece of art.
- Spend a few minutes seeing the object closely, noticing details you might not have seen before.
- Try to let go of any judgments or thoughts about the object and simply see it.

6. GUIDED MEDITATION:

- Listen to guided meditation recordings or apps that lead you through mindfulness exercises. These often include body scans, relaxation, and breathing techniques.

7. MINDFUL JOURNALING:

- Write in a journal about your thoughts, emotions, and experiences without judgment. Use it as a tool for self-reflection and self-compassion.

8. MINDFUL DAILY ACTIVITIES:

- Incorporate mindfulness into everyday tasks, such as washing dishes, taking a shower, or brushing your teeth. Pay attention to the sensations, smells, and movements involved in these activities.

9. *LOVING-KINDNESS MEDITATION (METTA):*

- Send good wishes and positive intentions to yourself and others. Start with yourself, then move on to loved ones, acquaintances, and even those with whom you have conflicts.

10. Mindful Breathing Breaks: - Take short breaks during the day to focus on your breath for a few minutes. This can help reduce stress and improve focus.

11. Mindfulness in Daily Life: - Practice being fully present in your daily activities, whether it is listening attentively in conversations, being fully engaged in work, or enjoying a meal without distractions.

Regular practice of mindfulness techniques can help you become more aware of your thoughts and feelings, reduce anxiety, and stress, and improve your ability to respond to life's challenges in a calm and centered way. The key is to approach these exercises with an open, non-judgmental attitude and be patient with yourself as you develop your mindfulness skills.

Can you recommend a good meditation app?

Certainly! There are several excellent meditation apps available that offer a wide range of guided meditation sessions, mindfulness exercises, and relaxation techniques. Here are some popular meditation apps that you can consider:

1. *HEADSPACE:*

   - Headspace offers a variety of guided meditation sessions, including mindfulness, stress reduction, and sleep meditation. It is known for its user-friendly interface and structured meditation programs.

2. *CALM:*

   - Calm supplies guided meditations, sleep stories, breathing exercises, and relaxation music. It is designed to help with stress reduction, sleep improvement, and overall well-being.

3. *INSIGHT TIMER:*

   - Insight Timer offers a vast library of free guided meditations and mindfulness practices. It also includes a customizable timer for silent meditation sessions.

4. *TEN PERCENT HAPPIER:*

   - Ten Percent Happier provides meditation and mindfulness content with a focus on making meditation approachable and practical. It offers courses, guided sessions, and expert interviews.

5. *BUDDHI:*

   - Buddhi is designed to integrate mindfulness into your daily life. It offers guided meditations for various activities, such as traveling, work, and sleep.

6. *SIMPLE HABIT:*

- Simple Habit supplies short, five-minute meditation sessions designed to fit into busy schedules. It covers a wide range of topics, including stress, sleep, and focus.

7. *SMILING MIND:*

- Smiling Mind is a mindfulness app designed for all ages, including children and adolescents. It offers age- appropriate meditation exercises and programs.

8. *BREATHE:*

- Breathe offers guided meditation sessions, sleep stories, and mindfulness exercises. It focuses on reducing stress, improving sleep, and enhancing overall mental well- being.

9. *AURA:*

- Aura offers personalized meditation and mindfulness recommendations based on your preferences and needs. It also includes a meditation journal for self- reflection.

10. *OMANI:*

- Omani supplies a wide variety of meditation and mindfulness content, including guided sessions, ambient sounds, and binaural beats for relaxation and focus.

Most of these apps offer both free and premium subscription options, so you can explore their content and features before deciding on a subscription. The best meditation app for you will depend on your specific preferences, goals, and the style of meditation that resonates

TELL ME MORE ABOUT THE BENEFITS OF MEDITATION.

Meditation offers a wide range of physical, mental, and emotional benefits. Regular practice of meditation has been shown to positively affect overall well-being and can be a valuable tool for improving various aspects of life. Here are some of the key benefits of meditation:

1. *STRESS REDUCTION:*

- Meditation is best known for its stress-reducing effects. It helps activate the body's relaxation response, reducing the production of stress hormones like cortisol. This can lead to a greater sense of calm and reduced feelings of stress and anxiety.

2. *IMPROVED EMOTIONAL WELL-BEING:*

- Meditation can enhance emotional regulation and resilience. It helps individuals become more aware of their emotions and develop healthier ways of responding to them. This can lead to an improved mood and a greater sense of emotional stability.

3. *ENHANCED CONCENTRATION AND FOCUS:*

- Meditation practices often involve the cultivation of concentration and mindfulness. Regular meditation can improve attention span, enhance concentration, and increase the ability to sustain focus on tasks.

4. *BETTER SLEEP:*

- Meditation can help with sleep problems, including insomnia. Mindfulness meditation and relaxation techniques can promote better sleep patterns and improve the quality of sleep.

5. *REDUCED SYMPTOMS OF ANXIETY AND DEPRESSION:*

- Studies have shown that meditation can be effective in reducing symptoms of anxiety and depression. It can provide individuals with tools to manage and alleviate these conditions.

6. *GREATER SELF-AWARENESS:*

- Meditation encourages self-reflection and self-awareness. It allows individuals to explore their thoughts, emotions, and behavior patterns, leading to a deeper understanding of themselves.

7. *PAIN MANAGEMENT:*

- Mindfulness meditation has been used as part of pain management programs. It can help individuals better cope with chronic pain and improve their pain tolerance.

8. *LOWER BLOOD PRESSURE:*

- Meditation has been associated with reduced blood pressure levels. This can contribute to better cardiovascular health and a reduced risk of heart disease.

9. *IMPROVED RELATIONSHIPS:*

- Mindfulness practices can enhance empathy, communication, and conflict resolution skills. This can lead to healthier and more satisfying interpersonal relationships.

10. Increased Resilience: - Meditation can improve resilience in the face of life's challenges. It helps individuals develop a more adaptive response to stressors and setbacks.

11. Greater Creativity: - Some meditation practices, such as mindfulness meditation, can enhance creative thinking and problem-solving by promoting an open and receptive mindset.

12. Spiritual Growth: - For those seeking a spiritual path, meditation can ease a deeper connection with one's inner self or higher consciousness.

13. Reduced Symptoms of Post-Traumatic Stress Disorder (PTSD): - Meditation, particularly mindfulness-based approaches, has been used as part of therapy for individuals with PTSD to help reduce symptoms and improve emotional regulation.

14. Enhanced Overall Well-Being: - Meditation promotes a sense of overall well-being, balance, and inner peace. It can lead to greater life satisfaction and a more positive outlook on life.

It is important to note that the benefits of meditation often become more pronounced with consistent practice over time. Different forms of meditation, such as mindfulness, loving-kindness, and transcendental meditation, offer numerous benefits and may be more suitable for different individuals and goals. To experience these benefits, it is essential to incorporate meditation into your daily or weekly routine and approach it with an open and non-judgmental attitude.

TELL ABOUT MINERALS THAT HELP THE BODY.

Minerals are essential nutrients that play crucial roles in various bodily functions. They are classified into two categories: microminerals and trace minerals, based on the amount the body needs. Here are some important minerals and their roles in maintaining good health:

MICROMINERALS:

1. **Calcium:**
   - Role: Essential for strong bones and teeth, muscle function, blood clotting, and nerve transmission.
   - Food Sources: Dairy products, leafy greens, fortified foods, and almonds.

2. *PHOSPHORUS:*

   - Role: Important for bone and teeth formation, energy metabolism, and DNA synthesis.
   - Food Sources: Meat, dairy, nuts, and whole grains.

3. *MAGNESIUM:*

   - Role: Involved in muscle and nerve function, bone health, energy production, and DNA replication.
   - Food Sources: Leafy greens, nuts, seeds, whole grains, and legumes.

4. *SODIUM:*

   - Role: Helps regulate fluid balance, nerve function, and muscle contractions.
   - Food Sources: Table salt, processed foods, and natural sources like celery and beets.

5. *POTASSIUM:*

- Role: Important for maintaining fluid balance, muscle contractions (including the heart), and nerve function.
- Food Sources: Bananas, potatoes, oranges, and spinach.

6. *CHLORIDE:*

- Role: Works with sodium to maintain fluid balance and aids in digestion as a component of stomach acid.
- Food Sources: Table salt and some vegetables.

TRACE MINERALS:

1. **Iron:**
   - Role: Essential for oxygen transport in the blood (as part of hemoglobin) and energy production.
   - Food Sources: Red meat, poultry, beans, spinach, and fortified cereals.

2. *ZINC:*

- Role: Necessary for immune function, wound healing, DNA synthesis, and taste perception.
- Food Sources: Meat, seafood, nuts, and dairy products.

3. *COPPER:*

- Role: Required for the formation of red blood cells, connective tissue, and enzymes involved in energy production.

- Food Sources: Organ meats, seafood, nuts, and whole grains.

4. *SELENIUM:*

    - Role: Acts as an antioxidant, helps regulate thyroid function, and supports the immune system.
    - Food Sources: Brazil nuts, seafood, meat, and whole grains.

5. *IODINE:*

    - Role: Essential for thyroid hormone production, which regulates metabolism.
    - Food Sources: Iodized salt, seafood, and dairy products.

6. *MANGANESE:*

    - Role: Important for bone formation, blood clotting, and the metabolism of carbohydrates, amino acids, and cholesterol.
    - Food Sources: Nuts, whole grains, beans, and leafy greens.

7. *FLUORIDE:*

    - Role: Supports dental health by preventing tooth decay and strengthening tooth enamel.
    - Food Sources: Drinking water in areas with fluoridation, toothpaste, and some seafood.

8. *CHROMIUM:*

- Role: Enhances the action of insulin, which helps regulate blood sugar levels.
- Food Sources: Whole grains, nuts, and broccoli.

9. *MOLYBDENUM:*

- Role: Involved in the metabolism of sulfur-containing amino acids and detoxification processes.
- Food Sources: Legumes, grains, and leafy vegetables.

10. *COBALT:*

- Role: A component of vitamin B12, which is essential for red blood cell formation and neurological function.
- Food Sources: Found in foods containing vitamin B12, primarily animal products.

These minerals are vital for maintaining proper bodily functions and overall health. A balanced diet that includes a variety of foods from different food groups can help ensure that you obtain the necessary minerals your body needs. However, it is important to consume them in proper amounts, as both deficiencies and excesses can have adverse effects on health. If you have specific concerns about your mineral intake or have a medical condition that affects mineral absorption or metabolism, consult with a healthcare provider or registered dietitian for personalized guidance.

WHAT ARE THE SYMPTOMS OF ZINC DEFICIENCY?

Zinc is an essential mineral that plays a crucial role in various bodily functions, including immune system function, wound healing, DNA synthesis, and growth and development. Zinc deficiency can lead to a range of symptoms and health issues. Common symptoms of zinc deficiency include:

1. **Weakened Immune System:** Individuals with zinc deficiency may be more susceptible to infections and illnesses, as zinc is essential for the proper functioning of the immune system.

2. **Delayed Growth and Development:** In children, zinc deficiency can lead to stunted growth, delayed sexual maturation, and impaired cognitive development.

3. **Skin Problems:** Zinc deficiency can result in various skin issues, including:

    - Delayed wound healing.

    - Acne and skin rashes

    - Dry and flaky skin

    - Hair loss or thinning

4. **Loss of Appetite and Weight Loss:** A lack of zinc can lead to a reduced sense of taste and smell, which can result in a loss of appetite and later weight loss.

5. **Gastrointestinal Problems:** Zinc is important for supporting the integrity of the gastrointestinal lining. Zinc deficiency can lead to diarrhea, abdominal pain, and impaired absorption of other nutrients.

6. **Impaired Sense of Taste and Smell:** One of the early signs of zinc deficiency is a diminished sense of taste and smell.

7. **Eye and Vision Problems:** Severe zinc deficiency may cause changes in the retina, leading to night blindness and other vision problems.

8. **Mood Disturbances:** Zinc plays a role in mood regulation, and deficiency may contribute to mood disturbances such as depression and irritability.

9. **Hair and Nail Changes:** Brittle nails and changes in hair texture, such as thinning or increased hair shedding, can be indicative of zinc deficiency.

10. **Neurological Symptoms:** Severe, long-term zinc deficiency can lead to neurological symptoms such as numbness and tingling in the extremities.

It's important to note that zinc deficiency is relatively uncommon in well-nourished individuals, but it can occur in certain populations at higher risk, such as vegetarians and vegans (as plant-based sources of zinc may be less bioavailable), individuals with gastrointestinal disorders that affect nutrient absorption, and those with increased zinc requirements, such as pregnant or lactating women.

If you suspect you have a zinc deficiency or are experiencing any of these symptoms, it is essential to consult with a healthcare professional for a proper evaluation and diagnosis. A healthcare provider can conduct blood tests to decide your zinc levels and recommend appropriate dietary changes or supplements if necessary. Self-diagnosis and self-treatment of mineral deficiencies can be risky and should be avoided.

Tell me more about zinc-rich foods.

Zinc is an essential mineral that plays a vital role in various bodily functions, including immune system function, wound healing, DNA synthesis, and the maintenance of healthy skin. Incorporating zinc-rich foods into your diet can help ensure you meet your daily zinc requirements. Here are some foods that are useful sources of zinc:

1. *ANIMAL-BASED SOURCES:*

   - **Red Meat:** Beef, lamb, and pork are among the richest sources of zinc. Lean cuts like sirloin and tenderloin provide higher concentrations of zinc.
   - **Poultry:** Chicken and turkey are useful sources of zinc, especially in the dark meat and skin.
   - **Seafood:** Seafood, particularly oysters, is exceptionally high in zinc. Other seafood options like crab, lobster, and shrimp also contain zinc.
   - **Dairy Products:** Dairy foods like milk, cheese, and yogurt provide zinc, with cheese being one of the better sources.
   - **Eggs:** Eggs contain moderate amounts of zinc, with the yolk containing more than the egg white.

2. *PLANT-BASED SOURCES:*

   - **Legumes:** Legumes like chickpeas, lentils, and beans (e.g., black beans, kidney beans) are good plant-based sources of zinc. Soaking and sprouting legumes can improve zinc absorption.

- **Nuts and Seeds:** Certain nuts and seeds contain zinc. Pumpkin seeds (pepitas), sunflower seeds, almonds, and cashews are notable examples.
- **Whole Grains:** Whole grains like wheat, rice, and oats contain some zinc, although they also contain phytates, which can inhibit zinc absorption. However, soaking, or fermenting grains can reduce phytate content.
- **Tofu and Tempeh:** Soy-based products like tofu and tempeh provide zinc and are popular among vegetarians and vegans.
- **Vegetables:** While vegetables generally contain lower amounts of zinc compared to animal-based sources, some like spinach, mushrooms, and peas provide modest amounts.

3. *FORTIFIED FOODS:*

- Some cereals and plant-based milk alternatives (e.g., almond milk, soy milk) are fortified with zinc to enhance their nutritional content.

It is important to note that the bioavailability of zinc can be influenced by factors such as dietary phytates, which are present in certain plant-based foods and can inhibit zinc absorption. To maximize zinc absorption, consider these tips:

- Combine zinc-rich foods with sources of vitamin C, as vitamin C can enhance zinc absorption.

- Soak, sprout, or ferment legumes and grains to reduce phytate content.
- Avoid excessive consumption of foods high in dietary phytates, such as unprocessed whole grains, nuts, and seeds, in the same meal as zinc-rich foods.

The recommended dietary allowance (RDA) for zinc varies by age, sex, and life stage but ranges from 8 to 11 milligrams per day for adults. It is essential to maintain a balanced diet that includes a variety of zinc-rich foods to meet your zinc needs. If you have specific dietary restrictions or concerns about zinc intake, consider consulting with a registered dietitian or healthcare provider for personalized guidance.

What are the symptoms of vitamin D deficiency?

Vitamin D deficiency can lead to a range of symptoms and health problems. Vitamin D is essential for various bodily functions, including bone health, immune system function, and the absorption of calcium. When the body lacks adequate vitamin D, it can result in the following symptoms and complications:

1. *BONE HEALTH ISSUES:*

   - **Bone Pain:** Vitamin D deficiency can cause bone and joint pain, often felt as a dull, achy discomfort. This pain can occur in the back, legs, or ribs.

- **Osteoporosis:** A lack of vitamin D can lead to reduced calcium absorption, which, over time, can weaken bones and increase the risk of fractures, particularly in older adults.

2. *MUSCLE WEAKNESS AND FATIGUE:*

    - Muscle weakness and general fatigue can be associated with vitamin D deficiency. This can lead to reduced physical strength and endurance.

3. *INCREASED SUSCEPTIBILITY TO INFECTIONS:*

    - Vitamin D plays a role in supporting the immune system. A deficiency may make you more vulnerable to infections, including respiratory infections.

4. *MOOD CHANGES AND DEPRESSION:*

    - Some studies suggest a link between vitamin D deficiency and mood disorders like depression. It is thought that vitamin D may influence the production of serotonin, a neurotransmitter associated with mood regulation.

5. *IMPAIRED WOUND HEALING:*

Vitamin D is involved in the wound healing process. A deficiency can lead to delayed wound healing and increased risk of infection at the wound site.

6. *HAIR LOSS:*

   - Excessive hair loss or thinning hair can be a symptom of vitamin D deficiency.

7. *MUSCLE CRAMPS AND PAIN:*

   - Muscle cramps and chronic muscle pain may occur in individuals with low vitamin D levels.

8. *COGNITIVE IMPAIRMENT:*

   - Some research suggests that vitamin D deficiency may be associated with cognitive decline and an increased risk of neurodegenerative diseases like Alzheimer's disease.

9. *DIGESTIVE PROBLEMS:*

   - Vitamin D is involved in calcium absorption, so deficiency can lead to digestive issues like diarrhea or irritable bowel syndrome (IBS).

10. *CARDIOVASCULAR HEALTH ISSUES:*

   - There is ongoing research exploring the potent deficiency and an increased risk of cardiovascular problems, including hypertension and heart disease.

11. *AUTOIMMUNE DISEASES:*

- Some autoimmune diseases, such as multiple sclerosis and type 1 diabetes, have been associated with lower vitamin D levels.

It is important to note that the symptoms of vitamin D deficiency can vary from person to person, and some individuals may not experience any noticeable symptoms, especially in the early stages of deficiency. To confirm a vitamin D deficiency, a blood test measuring the concentration of 25-hydroxyvitamin D is typically conducted by a healthcare provider.

If you suspect you have a vitamin D deficiency or are experiencing any of these symptoms, it is essential to consult with a healthcare professional for proper evaluation and diagnosis. Treatment typically involves vitamin D supplementation and dietary adjustments, and the appropriate dosage should be determined by a healthcare provider based on individual needs.

WHAT ARE THE BEST WAYS TO INCREASE VITAMIN D LEVELS?

Increasing vitamin D levels can be achieved through a combination of dietary changes, sun exposure, and, if necessary, supplementation. Here are some of the best ways to boost your vitamin D levels:

1. *SUN EXPOSURE:*

- The most natural way to increase vitamin D levels is through sunlight exposure. When your skin is exposed to UVB rays from sunlight, it can produce vitamin D. Spend some time outdoors in direct sunlight, without sunscreen, during the midday hours when the sun is at its strongest.
- The amount of sunlight needed varies based on factors like your skin tone, location, and time of year. Generally, 10-30 minutes of sun exposure to your arms, legs, face, and back several times a week is sufficient. Be cautious not to overexpose your skin to prevent sunburn.

2. VITAMIN D-RICH FOODS:

- Include foods high in vitamin D in your diet. Some good dietary sources of vitamin D include:
    - Fatty fish like salmon, mackerel, and trout
    - Cod liver oil
    - Fortified foods like milk, orange juice, and breakfast cereals
    - Eggs (particularly the yolks)
    - Cheese
    - Beef liver

3. SUPPLEMENTS:

- If you have a vitamin D deficiency or have difficulty obtaining enough through sunlight and diet, your healthcare provider may recommend vitamin D supplements. These are available in various forms, including vitamin D2 and vitamin D3. Vitamin D3 (cholecalciferol) is generally considered more effective at raising blood levels of vitamin D.

4. *UVB LAMPS:*

- Some people with specific medical conditions or those in regions with limited sunlight exposure may benefit from using UVB lamps. These lamps emit UVB radiation, which can stimulate vitamin D production in the skin.

5. *FORTIFIED FOODS:*

- Incorporate fortified foods into your diet. Many food products, including dairy alternatives like almond milk and soy milk, are fortified with vitamin D. Check labels for added vitamin D content.

6. *DIETARY CHANGES:*

- Include more vitamin D-rich foods in your diet, as mentioned above.
- Consider consuming foods that support vitamin D absorption, such as those high in dietary fats (since vitamin D is fat-soluble) and foods containing magnesium.

7. *REGULAR BLOOD TESTS:*

- If you are concerned about your vitamin D levels or have specific health conditions, consult with your healthcare provider, and request a blood test to measure your serum 25- hydroxyvitamin D levels. This test can help determine if you have a deficiency.

8. *BE MINDFUL OF FACTORS AFFECTING ABSORPTION:*

- Some factors can affect vitamin D absorption. These include obesity, age, certain medical conditions (like celiac disease or Crohn's disease), and certain medications. If you have these risk factors, consult with a healthcare provider to determine your vitamin D needs.

It is important not to overdo it with vitamin D supplements, as excessive intake can lead to toxicity. It is generally recommended to follow your healthcare provider's advice and dosing recommendations if you are considering vitamin D supplementation. Additionally, remember that maintaining a balanced diet and overall healthy lifestyle can contribute to better overall vitamin D status and overall health.

Covid 19 remedies like Ivermectin

2 / 2

As of my last knowledge update in September 2021, the use of Ivermectin for the prevention or treatment of COVID-19 had generated significant debate and controversy within the medical and scientific communities. It is important to note that the situation regarding COVID-19 treatments and research may have evolved since that time.

Here are some key points regarding Ivermectin and its use in relation to COVID-19:

1. **Lack of Definitive Evidence:** As of my last update, there was limited high-quality, peer-reviewed clinical evidence to support the use of Ivermectin as a COVID-19 treatment or prevention.

method. While some studies suggested potential benefits, others found no significant impact on COVID-19 outcomes.

2. **Guidance from Health Authorities:** Major health organizations, including the World Health Organization (WHO), the U.S. Food and Drug Administration (FDA), and the National Institutes of Health (NIH), had not recommended Ivermectin as a standard treatment or prevention measure for COVID-19. They emphasized the importance of relying on treatments that had undergone rigorous testing in clinical trials.

3. **Safety Concerns:** Ivermectin can have side effects, and the misuse or overuse of this medication can lead to adverse reactions, including nausea, vomiting, diarrhea, dizziness, and even more severe neurological effects in some cases. High doses or misuse of Ivermectin can be dangerous.

4. **Ongoing Research:** Research on potential treatments for COVID-19 continues to evolve, and innovative studies may have emerged since my last update. It is crucial to rely on up- to-date information from trusted sources, such as health authorities and reputable scientific journals, when considering COVID-19 treatments.

5. **Consultation with Healthcare Providers:** If you have COVID-19 or are concerned about COVID-19 prevention, it is essential to consult with a healthcare provider for guidance. They can provide information about approved treatments, vaccines, and preventive measures based on the latest scientific evidence and guidelines.

Given the rapidly changing nature of the COVID-19 pandemic and the evolving research landscape, I recommend staying informed about the latest developments by referring to trusted sources such as and your local health department for guidance on COVID-19 prevention and treatment. Additionally, consult with healthcare professionals for personalized advice and treatment options.

What is a lovely home remedy for diabetes?

Managing diabetes typically requires a combination of lifestyle changes, including a healthy diet, regular physical activity, and medication or insulin therapy under a healthcare provider. While there are no home remedies that can cure diabetes, some natural approaches may help improve blood sugar control and support overall health. It is important to note that these home remedies should complement, not replace, medical advice and treatment. Always consult with a healthcare provider for personalized guidance on managing diabetes. Here are some home remedies and lifestyle tips for diabetes management:

1. *DIETARY MODIFICATIONS:*

   - **Balanced Diet:** Focus on a well-balanced diet that includes a variety of whole foods like fruits, vegetables, whole grains, lean proteins, and healthy fats.
   - **Carbohydrate Management:** Monitor your carbohydrate intake and choose complex carbohydrates with a low glycemic index (GI) to help stabilize blood sugar levels. Limit refined sugars and processed foods.
   - **Fiber-Rich Foods:** Incorporate fiber-rich foods like beans, lentils, oats, and vegetables into your meals. Fiber can

help slow the absorption of glucose and improve blood sugar control.

- **Portion Control:** Be mindful of portion sizes to avoid overeating, which can lead to spikes in blood sugar levels.
- **Regular Meal Timing:** Try to eat meals and snacks at consistent times each day to help regulate blood sugar.

2. *PHYSICAL ACTIVITY:*

- Engage in regular physical activity, as exercise can help improve insulin sensitivity and lower blood sugar levels. Aim for at least 150 minutes of moderate-intensity aerobic activity per week, as recommended by health guidelines.

3. *WEIGHT MANAGEMENT:*

- Achieving and maintaining a healthy weight can help improve blood sugar control. Losing excess weight, even a modest amount, can have a positive impact on diabetes management.

4. *HYDRATION:*

- Stay well-hydrated with water, as it can help regulate blood sugar levels.

5. *STRESS REDUCTION:*

- Chronic stress can affect blood sugar control. Practice stress-reduction techniques such as deep breathing, meditation, yoga, or mindfulness to manage stress levels.

6. *HERBAL SUPPLEMENTS:*

- Some herbal supplements, like cinnamon and fenugreek, have been studied for their potential benefits in improving blood sugar control. Consult with a healthcare provider before using herbal remedies, as they may interact with medications.

7. *REGULAR MONITORING:*

- Monitor your blood sugar levels regularly as advised by your healthcare provider. This will help you track your progress and make necessary adjustments to your treatment plan.

8. *LIMIT ALCOHOL AND QUIT SMOKING:*

- If you consume alcohol, do so in moderation and with food. Quit smoking, as smoking can contribute to complications associated with diabetes.

9. *ADEQUATE SLEEP:*

- Prioritize good sleep hygiene to ensure you get enough quality sleep. Poor sleep can affect blood sugar levels and overall health.

10. *CONSULT A REGISTERED DIETITIAN:*

- Consider working with a registered dietitian who specializes in diabetes care. They can provide personalized dietary recommendations and guidance.

Remember that diabetes management should be tailored to your specific needs and may require medication or insulin therapy as prescribed by a healthcare provider. Always consult with a healthcare professional to create a comprehensive diabetes management plan that suits your individual circumstances.

top ten best vitamins and minerals

Vitamins and minerals are essential nutrients that play various critical roles in maintaining overall health and well-being. While the "best" vitamins and minerals can vary depending on an individual's specific needs, here are ten important vitamins and minerals that are generally considered essential for health:

1. *VITAMIN D:*

- Essential for bone health, immune system function, and overall well-being. It is often called the "sunshine vitamin" because the skin can produce it when exposed to sunlight.

2. *VITAMIN C (ASCORBIC ACID):*

- An antioxidant that supports the immune system, helps with wound healing, and aids in the absorption of iron from plant- based foods.

3. *VITAMIN A:*

- Necessary for vision, immune function, and skin health. It also plays a role in the health of the heart, lungs, and kidneys.

4. *VITAMIN K:*

- Essential for blood clotting and bone health. There are two main forms: K1 (found in leafy greens) and K2 (synthesized by gut bacteria and found in some fermented foods).

5. VITAMIN B12 (COBALAMIN):

- Important for nerve function, the formation of red blood cells, and DNA synthesis. It is primarily found in animal-based foods.

6. FOLATE (VITAMIN B9):

- Essential for cell division and the formation of DNA and RNA. It is particularly important during pregnancy to prevent neural tube defects in the fetus.

7. IRON:

- Crucial for transporting oxygen in the blood and for overall energy production. Iron deficiency can lead to anemia.

8. CALCIUM:

- Vital for bone and teeth health, muscle function, nerve signaling, and blood clotting.

9. MAGNESIUM:

- Involved in hundreds of biochemical reactions in the body, including muscle and nerve function, blood glucose control, and bone health.

10. Zinc: - Necessary for immune function, wound healing, and the synthesis of DNA. It also plays a role in taste perception and maintaining healthy skin.

These vitamins and minerals are essential for various bodily functions, and a balanced diet that includes a variety of foods can help ensure.

you get an adequate intake. It is important to note that the best way to obtain these nutrients is through a well-rounded and diverse diet. However, in some cases, supplementation may be necessary if you have specific deficiencies or dietary restrictions. Before taking any supplements, it is advisable to consult with a healthcare provider or registered dietitian to ensure that they are appropriate for your individual needs.

SKINCARE SUPPORT

Skincare is an important aspect of overall health and well-being. Proper skincare can help maintain healthy skin, prevent various skin issues, and promote a youthful appearance. Here are some tips and practices to support good skincare:

1. DAILY CLEANSING:

- Use a gentle cleanser to wash your face twice daily, typically in the morning and before bedtime. Choose a cleanser that suits your skin type (e.g., oily, dry, sensitive).

2. SUN PROTECTION:

- Protect your skin from the sun's harmful UV rays by wearing sunscreen with at least SPF 30 when you are outdoors. Reapply sunscreen every two hours, especially if you are swimming or sweating.
- Wear protective clothing like wide-brimmed hats and sunglasses to shield your face from the sun.

3. MOISTURIZE:

- Apply a moisturizer that suits your skin type to keep it hydrated. Dry skin can lead to flakiness and premature aging, while oily skin can still benefit from lightweight, non-comedogenic moisturizers.

4. *AVOID HARSH PRODUCTS:*

- Avoid using harsh soaps and skincare products that contain alcohol or synthetic fragrances, as these can strip the skin of natural oils and cause irritation.

5. *GENTLE EXFOLIATION:*

- Exfoliate your skin 1-2 times per week to remove dead skin cells and promote cell turnover. Choose a gentle exfoliant appropriate for your skin type.

6. *HYDRATION:*

- Drink plenty of water to keep your skin hydrated from within. Proper hydration can help maintain skin elasticity and a healthy complexion.

7. *BALANCED DIET:*

- Eat a balanced diet rich in fruits, vegetables, whole grains, lean proteins, and healthy fats. Nutrients like vitamins C and E, zinc, and omega-3 fatty acids are important for skin health.

8. *AVOID SMOKING AND LIMIT ALCOHOL:*

- Smoking can accelerate the aging process of the skin and lead to wrinkles and a dull complexion. Excessive alcohol consumption can dehydrate the skin.

9. *STRESS MANAGEMENT:*

- Chronic stress can exacerbate skin conditions like acne and eczema. Practice stress management techniques like meditation, deep breathing, or yoga.

10. Get Adequate Sleep: - Quality sleep is essential for skin repair and rejuvenation. Aim for 7-9 hours of restful sleep per night.

11. Skincare Routine: - Establish a consistent skincare routine that includes cleansing, toning, moisturizing, and sun protection. Tailor your routine to your skin's specific needs.

12. Consult a Dermatologist: - If you have specific skin concerns or conditions like acne, eczema, or psoriasis, consult a dermatologist for professional guidance and treatment options.

13. Avoid Touching Your Face: - Minimize touching your face, as this can transfer dirt and bacteria from your hands to your skin and potentially lead to breakouts.

14. Use Clean Makeup Brushes and Tools: - Regularly clean your makeup brushes and tools to prevent the buildup of bacteria and germs.

Remember that everyone's skin is unique, and what works for one person may not work for another. It is essential to tailor your skincare routine to your specific skin type and concerns. Additionally, be patient and consistent with your skincare practices, as it may take time to see noticeable improvements. If you have specific skin concerns or conditions, consider seeking advice from a skincare professional or dermatologist.

What are some natural remedies for stress?

Stress is a common part of life, but it is important to manage it effectively to maintain your overall well-being. Natural remedies for stress can help you relax, reduce tension, and promote a sense of calm. Here are some natural strategies to consider:

1. *DEEP BREATHING:*

    - Practice deep breathing exercises to activate the body's relaxation response. Take slow, deep breaths in through your nose, hold for a few seconds, and then exhale slowly through your mouth. Repeat several times.

2. *PROGRESSIVE MUSCLE RELAXATION (PMR):*

    - PMR involves systematically tensing and then relaxing different muscle groups in your body. This can help release physical tension associated with stress.

3. *MINDFULNESS MEDITATION:*

    - Mindfulness meditation involves focusing your attention on the present moment without judgment. Regular practice can reduce stress and improve emotional well- being.

4. *YOGA:*

    - Yoga combines physical postures, breathing techniques, and mindfulness to promote relaxation and reduce.

stress. Many styles of yoga are accessible for people of all fitness levels.

5. *AROMATHERAPY:*

- Certain scents, like lavender, chamomile, and rose, are known for their calming properties. You can use essential oils, candles, or diffusers to create a calming atmosphere.

6. *HERBAL TEAS:*

- Herbal teas like chamomile, valerian root, and passionflower have been used traditionally to promote relaxation and reduce stress.

7. *PHYSICAL ACTIVITY:*

- Regular exercise can help reduce stress hormones and trigger the release of endorphins, which are natural mood lifters. Activities like walking, jogging, swimming, or dancing can be effective.

8. *NATURE AND GREEN SPACES:*

- Spending time in nature or green spaces can have a calming effect on the mind and reduce stress. Even a short walk in a park can make a difference.

9. *LAUGHTER:*

- Laughter can release endorphins and reduce stress hormones. Watch a funny movie, spend time with friends who make you laugh, or engage in activities that bring you joy.

10. *SOCIAL SUPPORT:*

- Talking to friends and loved ones can provide emotional support during stressful times. Sharing your feelings and concerns can be therapeutic.

11. *LIMIT STIMULANTS:*

- Reduce or eliminate the consumption of caffeine and alcohol, which can exacerbate stress and anxiety in some individuals.

12. *HEALTHY DIET:*

- Consume a balanced diet rich in whole foods, fruits, vegetables, and lean proteins. Nutrient-rich foods can support overall well-being and stress management.

13. *SLEEP HYGIENE:*

- Prioritize good sleep habits by maintaining a regular sleep schedule, creating a comfortable sleep environment, and practicing relaxation techniques before bedtime.

14. *TIME MANAGEMENT:*

- Organize your tasks and priorities to reduce feelings of overwhelm. Break tasks into manageable steps and set realistic goals.

15. *LIMIT SCREEN TIME:*

- Reduce exposure to screens and electronic devices, especially before bedtime, as excessive screen time can contribute to stress and sleep disturbances.

It is essential to find the natural remedies and stress management techniques that work best for you. Keep in mind that stress is normal.

part of life, and it is not always possible to eliminate it entirely. However, by incorporating these natural strategies into your routine, you can better cope with stress and improve your overall well-being. If your stress becomes overwhelming or chronic, consider seeking support from a mental health professional or counselor.

Top twenty foods to avoid to better your health.

To improve your overall health, it is advisable to limit or avoid certain foods that are often associated with health risks when consumed in excess. Here are twenty foods to consider avoiding or consuming in moderation for better health:

1. **Sugar-Sweetened Beverages:** Sugary drinks like soda, fruit juices, and energy drinks are linked to obesity, type 2 diabetes, and dental problems.

2. **Processed Meats:** Processed meats like hot dogs, bacon, and sausages contain additives and preservatives and are associated with a higher risk of certain cancers and heart disease.

3. **Trans Fats:** Trans fats, often found in partially hydrogenated oils, are harmful to heart health. Avoid foods with hydrogenated or partially hydrogenated oils in the ingredient list.

4. **Fast Food:** Fast food items are typically high in unhealthy fats, sodium, and calories. Frequent consumption can contribute to weight gain and chronic health conditions.

5. **Fried Foods:** Fried foods are often high in unhealthy fats and can lead to weight gain and heart disease. opt for baked or grilled options when possible.

6. **Highly Processed Snacks:** Many packaged snacks like chips, cookies, and crackers are high in unhealthy fats, sugars, and additives. Choose healthier snack options like nuts, seeds, and whole fruits.

7. **Sugary Cereals:** Some breakfast cereals are loaded with added sugars. Look for cereals with minimal added sugars and high fiber content.

8. **Artificial Sweeteners:** While not all artificial sweeteners are harmful, excessive consumption may disrupt metabolism and appetite regulation. Moderation is key.

9. **Candy and Sweets:** Excessive consumption of candy and sweets can lead to weight gain, dental problems, and an increased risk of chronic diseases.

10. **White Bread and Pastries:** Foods made from refined white flour, such as white bread and pastries, have a high glycemic index and may contribute to blood sugar spikes.

11. **High-Sodium Foods:** Excessive sodium intake can increase blood pressure and the risk of heart disease. Limit foods like canned soups, processed meats, and salty snacks.

12. **Excessive Alcohol:** While moderate alcohol consumption may have some health benefits, excessive drinking can lead to various health issues, including liver disease and addiction.

13. **Sugary Breakfast Cereals:** Many sugary breakfast cereals are marketed to children and can lead to sugar cravings and unhealthy eating habits.

14. **Sugary Coffee Drinks:** Coffee beverages with excessive sugar and added syrups can contribute to excess calorie intake and blood sugar spikes.

15. **Highly Sweetened Yogurts:** Some flavored yogurts are high in added sugars. opt for plain yogurt and add your own fresh fruits for sweetness.

16. **Processed Cheese:** Highly processed cheese products often contain unhealthy additives and may not provide the same nutritional benefits as natural cheeses.

17. **Regular Potato Chips:** Potato chips are typically high in unhealthy fats and sodium. Consider healthier chip alternatives like baked vegetable chips.

18. **Deep-Fried Snacks:** Snacks like onion rings and fried mozzarella sticks are high in unhealthy fats and calories. Enjoy them sparingly.

19. **Margarine:** Some margarine products contain trans fats. Choose soft, trans-fat-free margarines or use healthier alternatives like olive oil.

20. **Excessive Fruit Juice:** While 100% fruit juice can provide some vitamins, it is also high in sugar. Limit consumption and prioritize whole fruits instead.

Remember that occasional indulgence in less healthy foods is okay, but it is essential to maintain a balanced diet rich in fruits, vegetables, lean proteins, and whole grains for overall health and well-being.

Moderation and portion control are key factors in maintaining a healthy diet. Additionally, dietary choices should be tailored to individual needs and health goals, so consulting with a registered dietitian or healthcare provider can provide personalized guidance.

More info on the foods to avoid.

Certainly, here is more detailed information about the foods to avoid or consume in moderation for better health:

1. **Sugar-Sweetened Beverages:** These include soda, fruit juices, energy drinks, and sweetened iced teas. They are high in added sugars, which can lead to weight gain, insulin resistance, and an increased risk of type 2 diabetes and heart disease.

2. **Processed Meats:** These are meats that have undergone processes like curing, smoking, or adding preservatives. Examples include hot dogs, sausages, and bacon. Processed meats are linked to an increased risk of colorectal cancer and heart disease.

3. **Trans Fats:** Trans fats are artificially created fats found in partially hydrogenated oils. They raise LDL (bad) cholesterol levels and increase the risk of heart disease. Food labels may list them as hydrogenated or partially hydrogenated oils.

4. **Fast Food:** Fast food items are often high in unhealthy fats, sodium, and calories. Frequent consumption can contribute to obesity, high blood pressure, and other health issues.

5. **Fried Foods:** Foods deep-fried in unhealthy oils are high in calories and saturated fats. Regular consumption can lead to weight gain, heart disease, and high cholesterol.

6. **Highly Processed Snacks:** Snacks like chips, cookies, and crackers are typically loaded with unhealthy fats, sugars, sodium, and artificial additives. These contribute to weight gain and poor nutritional intake.

7. **Sugary Cereals:** Many cereals marketed to children contain elevated levels of added sugars, which can lead to energy spikes and crashes and may contribute to weight gain.

8. **Artificial Sweeteners:** While artificial sweeteners can be useful for some, excessive consumption may disrupt metabolism and lead to increased sugar cravings. It is essential to use them in moderation.

9. **Candy and Sweets:** These items are often packed with added sugars and offer little to no nutritional value. Overconsumption can lead to obesity, dental issues, and chronic health problems.

10. **White Bread and Pastries:** Foods made from refined white flour, such as white bread and pastries, are low in fiber and nutrients. They can cause rapid spikes in blood sugar levels.

11. **High-Sodium Foods:** Excessive sodium intake can contribute to high blood pressure and increase the risk of stroke, heart disease, and kidney problems. Processed foods, canned soups, and salty snacks are common sources of high sodium.

12. **Excessive Alcohol:** While moderate alcohol consumption may have some health benefits, excessive drinking can lead to liver.

damage, addiction, accidents, and an increased risk of certain cancers.

13. **Sugary Breakfast Cereals:** Many sugary cereals are marketed to children and can lead to increased sugar cravings and unhealthy eating habits. They often lack essential nutrients.

14. **Sugary Coffee Drinks:** Coffee beverages loaded with sugar, syrups, and whipped cream can contain a day's worth of calories and sugar in a single cup. They can contribute to weight gain and blood sugar spikes.

15. **Highly Sweetened Yogurts:** Flavored yogurts are often high in added sugars. Choose plain yogurt and add fresh fruits or honey for sweetness.

16. **Processed Cheese:** Highly processed cheese products can contain unhealthy additives and may lack the nutritional benefits of natural cheeses. opt for natural cheese options when possible.

17. **Regular Potato Chips:** These snacks are typically fried in unhealthy oils and loaded with sodium. They can contribute to weight gain and high blood pressure.

18. **Deep-Fried Snacks:** Snacks like fried mozzarella sticks and onion rings are high in unhealthy fats and calories. Consuming them frequently can lead to weight gain and heart issues.

19. **Margarine:** Some margarine products contain trans fats, which are unhealthy for heart health. Choose margarine products that are free of trans fats or use healthier alternatives like olive oil.

20. **Excessive Fruit Juice:** While 100% fruit juice can provide some vitamins, it is also high in sugar and lacks the fiber found in whole fruits. Limit consumption and prioritize whole fruits for better health.

It is important to remember that while these foods should be limited, occasional indulgence is okay. A balanced diet rich in whole foods, including fruits, vegetables, lean proteins, and whole grains, should be the foundation of a healthy eating plan. Additionally, individual dietary choices should consider personal health goals and dietary restrictions, so consulting with a registered dietitian or healthcare provider for personalized guidance is recommended.

Tell me more about healthy snacks.

Healthy snacks can be an essential part of a balanced diet, providing nourishment between meals and helping to maintain energy levels throughout the day. The key to choosing healthy snacks is to opt for options that are nutritious, satisfying, and contribute to your overall well-being. Here are some ideas and guidelines for healthy snacking:

1. *FRUITS:*

   - Fresh fruits like apples, bananas, berries, and citrus fruits are excellent snack choices. They provide vitamins, minerals, fiber, and natural sweetness. Pair them with a small amount of nut butter or yogurt for added protein and satiety.

2. *VEGETABLES:*

- Raw vegetables like carrot sticks, celery, cucumber, and cherry tomatoes are low in calories and high in fiber. Dip them in hummus or a Greek yogurt-based dip for extra flavor and protein.

3. *NUTS AND SEEDS:*

    - Almonds, walnuts, pistachios, and pumpkin seeds are nutrient-dense snacks rich in healthy fats, protein, and fiber. Keep portions in check (about a small handful) to manage calorie intake.

4. *GREEK YOGURT:*

    - Greek yogurt is an excellent source of protein and probiotics, which support gut health. Top it with fresh fruit, honey, or a sprinkle of granola for added flavor and texture.

5. *NUT BUTTER:*

    - Nut butters like almond butter or peanut butter (preferably without added sugars or oils) can be spread on whole-grain crackers, apple slices, or whole-grain toast.

6. *HUMMUS:*

    - Hummus, made from chickpeas, provides protein and fiber. Enjoy it with whole-grain pita bread, carrot sticks, or cucumber slices.

7. *COTTAGE CHEESE:*

- Cottage cheese is a protein-rich snack option. Top it with fruit, a drizzle of honey, or a sprinkle of cinnamon for a sweet and savory combination.

8. *HARD-BOILED EGGS:*

- Hard-boiled eggs are a convenient source of protein and healthy fats. Sprinkle them with a pinch of salt and pepper for extra flavor.

9. *TRAIL MIX:*

- Make your own trail mix by combining a variety of nuts, seeds, and dried fruits. Be mindful of portion sizes to avoid excessive calorie intake.

10. *WHOLE-GRAIN SNACKS:*

- opt for whole-grain crackers, rice cakes, or whole-grain tortilla chips. These provide fiber and can be paired with healthy toppings like avocado or salsa.

11. *HOMEMADE SMOOTHIES:*

- Blend together Greek yogurt, fruits, and vegetables for a nutritious and satisfying smoothie. Avoid adding excessive sugar or sweeteners.

12. *LOW-FAT CHEESE:*

- Low-fat cheese, like string cheese or cheese cubes, can provide protein and calcium. Pair it with whole-grain crackers or apple slices.

13. *CHIA PUDDING:*

- Chia seeds soaked in milk or yogurt create a creamy pudding that is rich in fiber, healthy fats, and protein. Customize it with your favorite toppings like berries or nuts.

14. *POPCORN:*

- Air-popped popcorn is a whole-grain snack that is low in calories. Season it with a sprinkle of nutritional yeast, herbs, or spices for flavor.

15. *FROZEN GRAPES:*

- Frozen grapes are a refreshing and naturally sweet snack. They can satisfy your sweet tooth without added sugars.

When choosing healthy snacks, aim to strike a balance between macronutrients (carbohydrates, protein, and fats) to keep you satisfied and provide sustained energy. Also, pay attention to portion sizes to avoid overeating. Snacking can be a beneficial part of your diet when you make mindful choices that align with your health goals.

Tell me more about healthy fats.

Healthy fats, also known as unsaturated fats, are an essential part of a balanced diet and play a crucial role in maintaining overall health. Unlike saturated fats and trans fats, which are associated with health risks when consumed in excess, healthy fats offer numerous health benefits. Here is more information about healthy fats and their sources:

TYPES OF HEALTHY FATS:

There are two main types of healthy fats:

1. *MONOUNSATURATED FATS:*

   - Monounsaturated fats are liquid at room temperature and can help reduce bad cholesterol levels while increasing good cholesterol levels in the blood.
   - Food sources: Olive oil, avocado, nuts (such as almonds, peanuts, and cashews), and seeds (like flaxseeds and pumpkin seeds) are rich in monounsaturated fats.

2. *POLYUNSATURATED FATS:*

   - Polyunsaturated fats are also liquid at room temperature and include essential fatty acids that the body needs but cannot produce on its own.
   - Two essential types of polyunsaturated fats are omega-3 and omega-6 fatty acids, both of which have unique health benefits.
   - Omega-3 fatty acids are known for their anti-inflammatory properties and are linked to heart and brain health.
   - Food sources: Fatty fish (salmon, mackerel, sardines), walnuts, flaxseeds, chia seeds, and soybean oil are excellent sources of polyunsaturated fats, especially omega-3 fatty acids.

HEALTH BENEFITS OF HEALTHY FATS:

1. **Heart Health:** Healthy fats can help reduce the risk of heart disease by improving cholesterol levels, reducing inflammation, and supporting overall cardiovascular health.

2. **Brain Health:** Omega-3 fatty acids, in particular, play a vital role in brain development and function. They are associated with improved cognitive function and a reduced risk of neurodegenerative diseases.

3. **Weight Management:** Including healthy fats in your diet can help you feel full and satisfied, which may reduce overeating and support weight management.

4. **Skin and Hair Health:** Healthy fats are essential for maintaining skin and hair health, as they contribute to moisture and overall appearance.

5. **Nutrient Absorption:** Fats are necessary for the absorption of fat- soluble vitamins (A, D, E, and K) and other fat-soluble nutrients in the body.

TIPS FOR INCORPORATING HEALTHY FATS:

- Use olive oil or avocado oil for cooking and salad dressings.

- Include fatty fish like salmon, trout, or mackerel in your diet at least twice a week.

- Snack on a handful of nuts or seeds for a satisfying and nutritious option.

- Spread natural nut butter on whole-grain toast or use it as a dip for fruits or vegetables.

- Add avocado slices to salads, sandwiches, or wraps.

- Choose whole foods like olives and fatty fruits over processed snacks.

While healthy fats offer numerous benefits, it is essential to consume them in moderation, as they are calorie dense. A balanced diet that includes a variety of foods, along with healthy fats, is key to promoting overall health and well-being. Additionally, it is essential to limit saturated and trans fats, which are found in many processed and fried foods, to maintain a healthy diet.

Tell me more about omega-3 fatty acids.

OMEGA-3 FATTY ACIDS ARE A TYPE OF POLYUNSATURATED FAT THAT IS ESSENTIAL FOR OVERALL HEALTH AND WELL-BEING. THESE FACTS ARE KNOWN FOR THEIR NUMEROUS HEALTH BENEFITS, PARTICULARLY IN SUPPORTING HEART HEALTH, BRAIN FUNCTION, AND REDUCING INFLAMMATION. THERE ARE THREE MAIN TYPES OF OMEGA-3 FATTY ACIDS THAT ARE COMMONLY DISCUSSED:

1. *ALPHA-LINOLENIC ACID (ALA):*

   - ALA is a type of omega-3 fatty acid found in plant- based sources.
   - Food sources: Flaxseeds, chia seeds, walnuts, hemp seeds, are rich in ALA.

2. *EICOSATETRAENOIC ACID (EPA):*

- EPA is a long-chain omega-3 fatty acid found primarily in fatty fish and certain seafood.
- Food sources: Fatty fish like salmon, mackerel, trout, sardines, and herring are excellent sources of EPA.

3. *DOCOSAHEXAENOIC ACID (DHA):*

- DHA is another long-chain omega-3 fatty acid, and it is also primarily found in fatty fish and seafood.
- Food sources: Fatty fish like salmon, mackerel, trout, sardines, and herring are rich in DHA.

HEALTH BENEFITS OF OMEGA-3 FATTY ACIDS:

1. **Heart Health:** Omega-3 fatty acids have been extensively studied for their positive impact on heart health. They can help reduce the risk of heart disease by:
   - Lowering triglyceride levels in the blood.
   - Reducing inflammation in the blood vessels.
   - Helping to prevent the formation of blood clots.
   - Improving blood vessel function and reducing blood pressure.
2. **Brain Health:** Omega-3 fatty acids are essential for proper brain development and function. DHA, in particular, is a major component of brain cell membranes and is crucial for cognitive function. It

- Support mood and reduce the risk of depression.

- Reduce the risk of age-related cognitive decline and neurodegenerative diseases like Alzheimer's disease.

3. **Inflammation and Immune System:** Omega-3 fatty acids have anti-inflammatory properties, which can help reduce chronic inflammation in the body. This is important because chronic inflammation is linked to various diseases, including heart disease, arthritis, and certain cancers.

4. **Eye Health:** DHA is also found in high concentrations in the retina of the eye, and it plays a role in maintaining eye health. Omega-3s may help reduce the risk of age-related macular degeneration (AMD) and dry eye syndrome.

5. **Pregnancy and Infant Development:** Omega-3s, especially DHA, are crucial during pregnancy for the development of the baby's brain and eyes. They are often recommended as a prenatal supplement.

DIETARY RECOMMENDATIONS:

- To reap the benefits of omega-3 fatty acids, it is advisable to include a variety of food sources in your diet. Fatty fish, such as salmon, mackerel, and sardines, are excellent choices.

- Plant-based sources like flaxseeds, chia seeds, and walnuts are good options for those following a vegetarian or vegan diet.

- Consider consulting with a healthcare provider or registered dietitian to determine whether omega-3 supplements are appropriate for your specific health needs, especially if you have heart disease, arthritis, or other health concerns.

Incorporating a variety of omega-3-rich foods into your diet can be a valuable step in promoting heart and brain health while reducing inflammation and supporting overall well-being.

Tell me more about sources of omega- 3s.

Omega-3 fatty acids are essential fats that offer numerous health benefits. They are categorized into three main types: alpha-linolenic acid (ALA), eicosatetraenoic acid (EPA), and docosahexaenoic acid (DHA). To ensure you are getting a well-rounded intake of omega-3s, it is helpful to include a variety of food sources. Here are common sources of omega-3 fatty acids:

1. *FATTY FISH:*

- Fatty fish are some of the best natural sources of EPA and DHA, the most beneficial forms of omega-3s.
- Examples of fatty fish: Salmon, mackerel, trout, sardines, herring, and anchovies.
- Aim to include fatty fish in your diet at least twice a week to meet your omega-3 needs.

2. *FLAXSEEDS:*

- Flaxseeds are rich in ALA, a type of omega-3 fatty acid. They are one of the most abundant plant-based sources of omega-3s.

- Ground flaxseeds are easier to digest and provide more nutritional benefits than whole flaxseeds.
- You can sprinkle ground flaxseeds on oatmeal, yogurt, smoothies, or use them as an egg substitute in baking recipes.

3. *CHIA SEEDS:*

- Chia seeds are another excellent plant-based source of ALA and provide fiber and essential nutrients.
- Add chia seeds to yogurt, oatmeal, or make chia seed pudding by mixing them with your choice of liquid (e.g., almond milk) and letting them soak until they form a gel-like consistency.

4. *WALNUTS:*

- Walnuts are a useful source of ALA and provide healthy fats, fiber, and antioxidants.
- Enjoy walnuts as a snack, sprinkle them on salads, or add them to oatmeal or yogurt.

5. *HEMP SEEDS:*

- Hemp seeds contain ALA and are also rich in protein, fiber, and essential minerals.
- You can sprinkle hemp seeds on salads, cereal, or blend them into smoothies.

6. *EDAMAME (SOYBEANS):*

- Edamame, young soybeans, are a source of ALA and provide protein and fiber.

- Steam or boil edamame and season with a little salt for a healthy snack or side dish.

7. *ALGAL OIL SUPPLEMENTS:*

- Algal oil supplements are derived from algae and provide a plant-based source of EPA and DHA, similar to what you find in fish oil.
- These supplements are a suitable option for vegetarians and vegans who want to increase their intake of omega-3s.

8. *COD LIVER OIL:*

- Cod liver oil is a supplement rich in both EPA and DHA. It is available in liquid or capsule form.
- It is an option for individuals who may not consume fish regularly but want to ensure adequate omega-3 intake.

9. *FORTIFIED FOODS:*

- Some foods, such as certain brands of milk, yogurt, eggs, and breakfast cereals, are fortified with omega-3s, typically in the form of ALA.
- Check food labels for information on omega-3 content and sources.

It is important to note that while plant-based sources of omega-3s (ALA) offer health benefits, they are not as potent as EPA and DHA from marine sources (fatty fish, algal oil). The body can convert some ALA into EPA and DHA, but this conversion is limited. Therefore, including both plant-based and marine sources of omega-3s in your diet can provide a well-rounded intake of these essential fatty acids and maximize their health benefits. If you have specific dietary preferences or restrictions, consider consulting with a registered dietitian for personalized guidance on meeting your omega-3 needs.

How much water a day is recommended to drink.

The recommended daily water intake can vary depending on several factors, including age, sex, activity level, climate, and overall health. However, a general guideline is to aim for about eight cups (64 ounces) of water per day for most adults. This is often referred to as the "8x8 rule."

Here are some factors to consider:

1. **Individual Needs:** Some people may require more or less water depending on factors like body size, metabolism, and activity level. Athletes and individuals in hot or humid climates, for example, may need more water to stay properly hydrated.

2. **Age:** The water needs of children, older adults, and infants can differ from those of young and middle-aged adults. Consult with a healthcare provider for specific recommendations.

3. **Health Conditions:** Certain medical conditions, such as kidney disease or heart conditions, may require adjustments to daily water intake. Follow your healthcare provider's guidance in such cases.

4. **Pregnancy and Breastfeeding:** Pregnant and breastfeeding women typically require more water to support the needs of their growing baby and milk production. Adequate hydration is crucial during these periods.

5. **Thirst:** Listen to your body's signals. The first is a natural indicator that your body needs more fluids. Pay attention to your thirst cues and drink water when you feel thirsty.

6. **Diet:** The foods you eat also contribute to your daily fluid intake. Fruits, vegetables, soups, and beverages other than water can provide additional hydration.

7. **Climate:** Hot and dry climates can lead to increased sweating and higher water loss, requiring more fluid intake to stay hydrated.

8. **Activity Level:** Physical activity increases your fluid requirements. Be sure to drink water before, during, and after exercise to stay hydrated.

While the "8x8 rule" is a simple guideline to follow, it is essential to adjust your water intake based on your individual circumstances. To monitor your hydration, pay attention to the color of your urine. Pale yellow or straw-colored urine indicates proper hydration, while dark yellow or amber-colored urine may suggest dehydration.

It is worth noting that thirst is a reliable indicator of when to drink water for most people. Drinking water when you are thirsty is a natural and effective way to meet your body's fluid needs. However, in certain situations, such as during strenuous exercise or in extreme heat, you may need to drink water even before you feel thirsty to prevent dehydration.

Ultimately, staying well-hydrated is essential for overall health, so it is important to be mindful of your fluid intake and adjust it as needed to meet your individual requirements.

What foods have high water content?

Many foods have high water content, which can contribute to your daily hydration needs. These foods are not only refreshing but also provide valuable vitamins, minerals, and dietary fiber. Including water-rich foods in your diet is a convenient way to help meet your daily fluid requirements. Here are some examples of foods with high water content:

1. **Cucumbers:** Cucumbers are made up of over 95% water, making them one of the most hydrating vegetables. They are refreshing and low in calories.

2. **Watermelon:** Watermelon is approximately 90% water and is a perfect summertime snack. It is also rich in vitamins A and C.

3. **Strawberries:** Strawberries are about 90% water and are packed with antioxidants, fiber, and vitamin C.

4. **Oranges:** Oranges have high water content, and they are an excellent source of vitamin C and other essential nutrients.

5. **Grapefruit:** Grapefruit is another citrus fruit with high water content. It is known for its tangy flavor and is rich in vitamins and minerals.

6. **Lettuce:** Most types of lettuce, such as iceberg and romaine, are composed of more than 90% water. They make a great base for salads.

7. **Celery:** Celery is crisp and refreshing, with a water content of over 95%. It is also a good source of fiber.

8. **Bell Peppers:** Bell peppers, especially the green variety, have a high-water content and are rich in vitamins A and C.

9. **Zucchini:** Zucchini is a summer squash with high water content and is versatile for cooking and grilling.

10. **Tomatoes:** Tomatoes are about 94% water and provide essential vitamins, particularly vitamin C and vitamin K.

11. **Radishes:** Radishes are crunchy and have a high-water content. They add a refreshing kick to salads.

12. **Pineapple:** Pineapple is a tropical fruit with a water content of approximately 86%. It is sweet and juicy and provides vitamin C and manganese.

13. **Cantaloupe:** Cantaloupe is rich in water, providing hydration along with vitamins A and C.

14. **Cabbage:** Cabbage varieties like green cabbage and red cabbage have a high-water content and are nutritious additions to coleslaw and salads.

15. **Berries:** Other than strawberries, berries like blueberries, raspberries, and blackberries also contain significant water content and are full of antioxidants.

16. **Apples:** Apples are made up of about 86% water and provide dietary fiber and various vitamins and minerals.

17. **Peaches:** Peaches are juicy and have a water content of around 89%. They are a useful source of vitamins A and C.

18. **Broccoli:** Broccoli is not as high in water content as some other vegetables but still provides hydration along with essential nutrients.

19. **Spinach:** Spinach contains over 90% water and is packed with vitamins, minerals, and antioxidants.
20. **Cauliflower:** Cauliflower has a moderate water content and is versatile for roasting, mashing, or using as a low-carb rice substitute.

Including these water-rich foods in your diet can help you stay hydrated and meet your daily fluid needs, especially on hot days or during periods of physical activity. Remember that water-rich foods complement your overall fluid intake, but you should still drink water regularly to maintain proper hydration.

Tell me more about vitamin C sources.

Vitamin C, also known as ascorbic acid, is a water-soluble vitamin that plays a crucial role in various bodily functions, including immune support, collagen production, and antioxidant protection. It is essential to obtain an adequate amount of vitamin C through your diet since the body cannot produce it on its own. Here are some common sources of vitamin C:

1. *CITRUS FRUITS:*

    - Oranges, lemons, limes, and grapefruits are well-known for their high vitamin C content. They are not only delicious but also provide a sizable portion of your daily vitamin C needs.

2. *BERRIES:*

- Berries like strawberries, blueberries, raspberries, and blackberries are excellent sources of vitamin C. They are also rich in antioxidants and other beneficial nutrients.

3. *KIWI:*

- Kiwifruit is packed with vitamin C and provides more vitamin C per serving than many other fruits. It is also a good source of dietary fiber and vitamin K.

4. *PINEAPPLE:*

- Pineapple is another tropical fruit that contains a considerable amount of vitamin C. It is a refreshing and sweet option.

5. *MANGO:*

- Mangoes are not only delicious but also rich in vitamins. C. They also provide vitamin A and dietary fiber.

6. *PAPAYA:*

- Papaya is known for its vitamin C content and is a useful source of vitamin A and folate. It has a sweet and tropical flavor.

7. *GUAVA:*

- Guava is one of the fruits with the highest vitamin C content. It is exceptionally rich in this vitamin and provides other nutrients like dietary fiber.

8. *CANTALOUPE:*

- Cantaloupe, a type of melon, contains vitamin C and is a hydrating fruit. It is also a good source of vitamin A.

9. *RED AND GREEN BELL PEPPERS:*

- Bell peppers, especially the red and green varieties, are excellent vegetable sources of vitamin C. Red bell peppers tend to have a higher vitamin C content than green ones.

10. *BROCCOLI:*

- Broccoli is a cruciferous vegetable that contains vitamin C along with other essential nutrients like fiber and vitamin K.

11. *CAULIFLOWER:*

- Cauliflower is another cruciferous vegetable with a notable vitamin C content. It is versatile for various culinary uses.

12. *SPINACH:*

- Spinach contains vitamin C and is a rich source of other vitamins, minerals, and antioxidants.

13. *KALE:*

- Kale is a leafy green vegetable that provides vitamin C, vitamin K, and other nutrients.

14. *TOMATOES:*

- Tomatoes are a source of vitamin C, particularly when consumed in their raw form. They are also rich in the antioxidant lycopene.

15. *POTATOES:*

- Potatoes, especially when consumed with the skin, provide vitamin C along with dietary fiber and potassium.

16. **Strawberry Kiwi:** A combination of strawberries and kiwifruit makes a vitamin C powerhouse. You can create delicious smoothies or fruit salads with these fruits.

17. *ACEROLA CHERRIES:*

- Acerola cherries are one of the richest sources of vitamin C, containing significantly higher levels than citrus fruits.

18. *BLACK CURRANTS:*

- Black currants are a lesser-known source of vitamin C, but they are quite rich in this vitamin.

19. *ROSE HIPS:*

- Rose hips, the fruit of the rose plant, are known for their high vitamin C content. They are often used to make herbal teas.

20. *SUPPLEMENTS:*

- In some cases, healthcare professionals may recommend vitamin C supplements to address specific deficiencies or health concerns.

It is important to include a variety of these vitamin C-rich foods in your diet to ensure you receive a broad range of nutrients along with vitamins.

C. Remember that vitamin C is sensitive to heat and can degrade during cooking, so consuming some of these foods raw or lightly cooked. can help preserve their vitamin C content.

Tell me more about vitamin D sources.

Vitamin D is a fat-soluble vitamin that is crucial for various bodily functions, including calcium absorption, bone health, immune system support, and cell growth. Unlike many other vitamins, vitamin D can be synthesized by the body when the skin is exposed to sunlight. However, it is also important to obtain vitamin D from dietary sources when sunlight exposure is limited. Here are common sources of vitamin D:

1. **Sunlight:** The sun is a natural source of vitamin D, and the body can synthesize it when the skin is exposed to ultraviolet B (UVB) rays. Sunlight exposure, especially during the midday hours, is the most effective way for the body to produce vitamin D.

Factors such as skin type, geographical location, season, and the use of sunscreen can influence the amount of vitamin D produced through sun exposure.

2. **Fatty Fish:** Fatty fish are among the best dietary sources of vitamin D. They naturally contain vitamin D3 (cholecalciferol), the same form synthesized by the skin when exposed to sunlight.

   - Examples of vitamin D-rich fish: Salmon, mackerel, trout, sardines, tuna, and cod liver oil.

3. **Egg Yolks:** Egg yolks are a source of vitamin D, although the amount can vary depending on the diet of the chickens. Eggs from chickens that are fed a diet rich in vitamin D will have higher vitamin D content.

4. **Fortified Foods:** Many foods are fortified with vitamin D to help people meet their daily requirements, especially when sunlight exposure is limited. These include:

   - Fortified dairy products (milk, yogurt, cheese).

   - Fortified plant-based milk alternatives (soy milk, almond milk, coconut milk).

   - Fortified breakfast cereals.

   - Fortified orange juice.

   - Fortified tofu.

   - Fortified margarine.

5. **Mushrooms:** Some types of mushrooms, such as shiitake and maitake mushrooms, naturally contain vitamin D2 (ergocalciferol), a plant-based form of the vitamin. Exposing

mushrooms to sunlight or ultraviolet (UV) light can increase their vitamin D content.

6. **Supplements:** Vitamin D supplements are available in various forms, including vitamin D2 and vitamin D3. These supplements can be an effective way to ensure you meet your vitamin D needs, especially if you have limited sun exposure or dietary restrictions.

It is important to note that vitamin D is a fat-soluble vitamin, which means it is better absorbed when consumed with dietary fats. Therefore, consuming vitamin D-rich foods with healthy fats, such as those found in fatty fish, avocado, nuts, and olive oil, can enhance its absorption.

The recommended daily intake of vitamin D can vary depending on age, sex, and life stage. If you have concerns about your vitamin D levels or are considering vitamin D supplements, it is advisable to consult with a healthcare provider or registered dietitian for personalized guidance based on your individual needs and circumstances. Additionally, some individuals, such as those with certain medical conditions or at-risk populations, may require higher vitamin D intake or specific supplementation recommendations.

Tell me more about vitamin K sources.

Vitamin K is a fat-soluble vitamin that plays a crucial role in blood clotting and bone health. There are two primary forms of vitamin K: vitamin K1 (phylloquinone) and vitamin K2 (menaquinone). Both forms are important for contrasting functions in the body. Here are common sources of vitamin K:

VITAMIN K1 SOURCES:

1. **Leafy Green Vegetables:** Leafy greens are some of the best sources of vitamin K1.
   - Examples: Spinach, kale, collard greens, Swiss chard, broccoli, Brussels sprouts, and parsley.
2. **Herbs:** Many herbs are rich in vitamin K1.
   - Examples: Basil, thyme, sage, and cilantro.
3. **Vegetables:** Some non-leafy vegetables also contain vitamin K1.
   - Examples: Green beans, asparagus, and okra.
4. **Fruits:** While fruits are not as high in vitamin K1 as vegetables, some contain lesser amounts.
   - Examples: Blueberries, grapes, and kiwi.
5. **Vegetable Oils:** Certain vegetable oils contain vitamin K1.
   - Examples: Soybean oil, canola oil, and olive oil.

VITAMIN K2 SOURCES:

1. **Fermented Foods:** Fermented foods are a natural source of vitamin K2.
   - Examples: Natto (fermented soybeans), sauerkraut, and fermented cheeses (such as Gouda and Brie).

2. **Meat and Animal Products:** Some animal-based foods contain vitamin K2, especially those from animals that have been grass- fed or pasture-raised.
   - Examples: Liver, chicken, ground beef, and egg yolks.

3. **Fatty Fish:** Certain fatty fish contain vitamin K2.
   - Examples: Salmon, mackerel, and sardines.

4. **Nuts and Seeds:** Some nuts and seeds provide vitamin K2.
   - Examples: Cashews, pistachios, and pumpkin seeds.

5. **Dairy Products:** Dairy products can contain lesser amounts of vitamin K2.
   - Examples: Cheese, particularly hard and soft cheeses like Gouda and Brie.

6. **Natto Supplements:** Natto supplements, which provide a concentrated source of vitamin K2 derived from fermented soybeans, are available for those who want to increase their vitamin K2 intake.

Vitamin K1 is primarily involved in blood clotting, while vitamin K2 plays a crucial role in regulating calcium metabolism, which is important for bone health and may have cardiovascular benefits. It is worth noting that vitamin K is also synthesized by the gut microbiota to some extent.

The recommended daily intake of vitamin K can vary depending on age, sex, and specific health needs. In general, a balanced diet that includes a variety of leafy greens, vegetables, fruits, fermented foods, and healthy fats can help you meet your vitamin K requirements. If you have specific concerns about vitamin K intake or are taking medications that affect vitamin K metabolism, it is advisable to consult.

with a healthcare provider or registered dietitian for personalized guidance.

Tell me more about vitamin E sources.

Vitamin E is a fat-soluble antioxidant that plays a crucial role in protecting cells from oxidative damage. It also supports immune function and skin health. There are several forms of vitamin E, but the most biologically active form is alpha tocopherol. Here are common sources of vitamin E:

1. **Nuts and Seeds:** Nuts and seeds are among the best dietary sources of vitamin E.

   - Examples: Almonds, sunflower seeds, hazelnuts, pine nuts, and peanuts.

2. **Vegetable Oils:** Vegetable oils are rich in vitamin E, particularly if they are unprocessed or minimally processed.

   - Examples: Sunflower oil, safflower oil, wheat germ oil, and olive oil.

3. **Leafy Green Vegetables:** Some leafy greens contain vitamin E, though they are not as high in vitamin E as nuts and seeds.

   - Examples: Spinach, Swiss chard, and turnip greens.

4. **Avocado:** Avocado is a source of vitamin E and is also rich in healthy fats and other nutrients.

5. **Fruits:** Some fruits supply vitamin E, although the levels are relatively low compared to other sources.
    - Examples: Kiwi, blackberries, and mangoes.

6. **Fortified Foods:** Certain breakfast cereals and food products are fortified with vitamin E to help individuals meet their daily requirements.

7. **Whole Grains:** Some whole grains contain vitamin E, albeit in smaller amounts compared to other sources.
    - Examples: Whole wheat, brown rice, and oats.

8. *SPINACH:*
    - Spinach is a leafy green vegetable that provides vitamin E along with other vitamins and minerals.

9. *BROCCOLI:*
    - Broccoli contains vitamin E and is a rich source of fiber and other nutrients.

10. *TOMATOES:*
    - Tomatoes provide a small amount of vitamin E and are also a source of antioxidants like lycopene.

11. *SHELLFISH:*
    - Some shellfish contain vitamin E, although the levels can vary.
    - Examples: Shrimp, crab, and lobster.

12. **Fatty Fish:** Fatty fish provide vitamin E along with heart-healthy omega-3 fatty acids.

- Examples: Salmon, mackerel, and trout.

It is important to note that vitamin E is found in various forms, including alpha-tocopherol, beta-tocopherol, gamma-tocopherol, and delta- tocopherol. Alpha-tocopherol is the most biologically active form and is often the focus of dietary recommendations.

A balanced diet that includes a variety of foods, especially those rich in healthy fats and antioxidants, can help you meet your vitamin E requirements. Keep in mind that vitamin E is sensitive to heat and oxygen, so minimizing processing and storage time of foods can help retain their vitamin E content. If you have specific dietary concerns or conditions that affect your vitamin E intake or absorption, consult with a healthcare provider or registered dietitian for personalized guidance.

Here are the benefits of vitamin E.

Vitamin E is an essential nutrient that offers a range of health benefits due to its antioxidant properties and its role in various bodily functions. Here are some of the key benefits of vitamin E:

1. **Antioxidant Protection:** Vitamin E is a powerful antioxidant that helps protect cells and tissues from oxidative damage caused by free radicals. This oxidative damage is associated with.

aging, chronic diseases, and the development of various health conditions.

2. **Skin Health:** Vitamin E is known for its positive effects on skin health. It can help moisturize and promote skin elasticity, reducing the appearance of fine lines and wrinkles. It is often found in skincare products and may help with wound healing and scar reduction.

3. **Heart Health:** Vitamin E may have cardiovascular benefits by helping to prevent the oxidation of low-density lipoprotein (LDL) cholesterol, often referred to as "bad" cholesterol. Oxidized LDL cholesterol is believed to contribute to the development of atherosclerosis (hardening of the arteries).

4. **Immune Support:** Vitamin E plays a role in supporting the immune system by helping immune cells function effectively. It can enhance the body's ability to fight off infections and diseases.

5. **Eye Health:** Vitamin E may have a protective effect against age-related eye conditions like cataracts and macular degeneration. It works in conjunction with other antioxidants like vitamin C and zinc to maintain eye health.

6. **Brain Health:** Some research suggests that vitamin E may help protect brain cells from oxidative stress, potentially reducing the risk of cognitive decline as people age. However, more studies are needed in this area.

7. **Anti-Inflammatory Effects:** Vitamin E has mild anti-inflammatory properties and may help reduce inflammation in the body. Chronic inflammation is linked to various diseases, so reducing inflammation can have long-term health benefits.

8. **Menstrual Pain Relief:** Some women find relief from menstrual cramps by taking vitamin E supplements, although individual responses may vary.

9. **Cancer Prevention:** While more research is needed, some studies suggest that vitamin E may play a role in reducing the risk of certain cancers, particularly prostate cancer.

10. **Hair Health:** Vitamin E can help improve hair health by promoting blood circulation in the scalp, which may contribute to healthier hair growth and reduced hair loss.

It is important to note that while vitamin E offers numerous health benefits, excessive supplementation of vitamin E supplements can be harmful and should be avoided unless recommended by a healthcare provider. In most cases, it is best to obtain vitamin E through a balanced diet that includes a variety of foods rich in this nutrient.

The recommended dietary allowance (RDA) for vitamin E varies by age and sex, so consult with a healthcare provider or registered dietitian to determine your specific vitamin E needs and the best ways to incorporate it into your diet for optimal health.

Here is me more about vitamin D deficiency.

Vitamin D deficiency occurs when a person's vitamin D levels fall below the recommended range, leading to potential health problems. Vitamin D is essential for various bodily functions, including.

calcium absorption, bone health, immune system support, and cell growth. Here is more information about vitamin D deficiency:

CAUSES OF VITAMIN D DEFICIENCY:

1. **Inadequate Sunlight Exposure:** The primary source of vitamin D for the body is sunlight. When the skin is exposed to UVB rays from the sun, it can produce vitamin D. Factors such as living in regions with limited sunlight, spending too much time indoors, or covering the skin can reduce sun exposure.

2. **Dietary Insufficiency:** A lack of dietary sources of vitamin D can contribute to deficiency. Few foods naturally contain significant amounts of vitamin D, and some people may have dietary restrictions that limit their intake of these foods.

3. **Malabsorption Issues:** Certain medical conditions, such as celiac disease, Crohn's disease, and other gastrointestinal disorders, can interfere with the absorption of vitamin D from the diet.

4. **Age:** As people age, their skin becomes less efficient at producing vitamin D from sunlight. Additionally, older individuals may have reduced dietary intake or limited exposure to sunlight.

5. **Obesity:** Vitamin D is a fat-soluble vitamin, and it can be sequestered in fat tissues. People with obesity may have lower bioavailability of vitamin D, even if they have sufficient dietary intake or sun exposure.

6. **Kidney and Liver Disorders:** Conditions that affect the kidneys or liver can impair the conversion of vitamin D into its active form, which is necessary for its biological functions.

Vitamin D deficiency can be asymptomatic (showing no obvious symptoms) in its preliminary stages. However, as deficiency worsens, various symptoms and health problems may develop, including:

1. **Bone Health Issues:** Vitamin D deficiency can lead to weakened bones, increased risk of fractures, and conditions like osteoporosis and osteoma Acia (softening of the bones).

2. **Muscle Weakness:** Vitamin D plays a role in muscle function, and deficiency can lead to muscle weakness and pain.

3. **Fatigue:** Some individuals with vitamin D deficiency report increased fatigue and a general lack of energy.

4. **Mood Changes:** There is a link between vitamin D deficiency and mood disorders like depression and Seasonal Affective Disorder (SAD).

5. **Impaired Immune Function:** Vitamin D is involved in immune system regulation, so deficiency may increase susceptibility to infections.

6. **Cognitive Impairment:** There is some evidence to suggest that low vitamin D levels are associated with cognitive decline and an increased risk of neurodegenerative diseases like Alzheimer's disease.

Prevention and Treatment:

Preventing and treating vitamin D deficiency typically involves increasing vitamin D intake through the following methods:

1. **Sunlight Exposure:** Spending time outdoors in the sun, especially during the midday hours, can help the skin produce vitamin D. However, it is important to balance sun exposure to avoid skin damage.

2. **Dietary Sources:** Consuming foods rich in vitamin D, such as fatty fish (salmon, mackerel), egg yolks, fortified dairy products, and fortified cereals, can help increase vitamin D intake.

3. **Supplements:** A healthcare provider may recommend Vitamin D supplements to correct a deficiency. The type and dose of supplements will depend on the individual's specific needs and health status.

If you suspect you have a vitamin D deficiency or are at risk, it is advisable to consult with a healthcare provider for proper evaluation, testing, and guidance on supplementation or dietary changes. Vitamin D deficiency is a common issue, but with appropriate intervention, it can often be effectively managed and prevented.

TELL ME MORE ABOUT VITAMIN K2.

Vitamin K2, also known as menaquinone, is one of the two primary forms of vitamin K, with the other being vitamin K1 (phylloquinone). While both forms are essential for various bodily functions, vitamin K2 is particularly known for its role in regulating calcium metabolism and supporting bone and cardiovascular health. Here is more information about vitamin K2:

TYPES OF VITAMIN K2:

There are several subtypes of vitamin K2, known as menaquinones (MKs), which vary in their structure and dietary sources. The most studied and biologically active forms of vitamin K2 are MK-4 and MK-7:

1. **MK-4:** This is a short-chain menaquinone and is found in animal- based foods, including meats, dairy products, and eggs. It is also synthesized from vitamin K1 in the body.

2. **MK-7:** This is a long-chain menaquinone and is primarily derived from fermented foods and certain bacteria in the gut. Fermented foods like natto (fermented soybeans) are particularly rich in MK-7.

FUNCTIONS OF VITAMIN K2:

Vitamin K2 has several essential functions in the body, including:

1. **Calcium Regulation:** One of the most well-known roles of vitamin K2 is in regulating calcium metabolism. It helps ensure that calcium is directed to the bones and teeth, where it is needed for strength, and away from soft tissues like blood vessels and kidneys, where excessive calcium deposition can lead to calcification and health issues.

2. **Bone Health:** Vitamin K2 plays a crucial role in maintaining bone health by activating a protein called osteocalcin, which is necessary for the proper mineralization of bone tissue. Adequate vitamin K2 intake may help reduce the risk of osteoporosis and fractures.

3. **Cardiovascular Health:** Some research suggests that vitamin K2 may support cardiovascular health by helping to prevent the

calcification of arteries. Arterial calcification is a risk factor for cardiovascular diseases like atherosclerosis.

4. **Dental Health:** Vitamin K2 may play a role in dental health by promoting the proper formation and mineralization of teeth.
5. **Anti-Inflammatory Properties:** Some studies suggest that vitamin K2 has anti-inflammatory properties, which can have a positive impact on overall health and reduce the risk of chronic diseases associated with inflammation.

Food Sources of Vitamin K2:

Dietary sources of vitamin K2 include:

1. **Fermented Foods:** Natto, a Japanese fermented soybean dish, is one of the richest sources of vitamin K2 (particularly MK-7). Other fermented foods like sauerkraut and certain cheeses also contain vitamin K2.
2. **Meat and Organ Meats:** Animal-based sources of vitamin K2 include liver, chicken, ground beef, and other meats.
3. **Dairy Products:** Dairy products like cheese and butter, especially when produced from grass-fed animals, contain vitamin K2.
4. **Egg Yolks:** Egg yolks from chickens raised on diets rich in vitamin K1 can provide some vitamin K2.

While vitamin K2 is important for health, it is also produced by some beneficial bacteria in the gut. A balanced diet that includes a variety of foods rich in both vitamin K1 and vitamin K2, along with a healthy gut microbiome, can contribute to overall vitamin K status.

As with any dietary component, it is essential to maintain a balanced diet and, if necessary, consult with a healthcare provider or registered dietitian to assess your specific vitamin K needs and whether supplementation is appropriate for your individual circumstances.

WHAT VITAMINS AND MINERALS SERVE THE IMMUNE SYSTEM THE BEST?

Several vitamins and minerals play important roles in supporting the immune system by helping it function effectively and efficiently. Here are some of the key vitamins and minerals that are known for their immune-boosting properties:

1. **Vitamin C:** Vitamin C is a potent antioxidant that helps protect immune cells from damage caused by free radicals. It also supports the production and function of white blood cells, which are essential for immune defense.
2. **Vitamin D:** Vitamin D is crucial for the proper functioning of the immune system. It helps regulate the production and activity of immune cells and plays a role in reducing inflammation. Adequate vitamin D levels are associated with a lower risk of respiratory infections.
3. **Vitamin A:** Vitamin A is essential for maintaining the health of mucous membranes, which are the body's first line of defense.

against pathogens. It also supports the production of immune cells and antibodies.

4. **Vitamin E:** Vitamin E is an antioxidant that helps protect immune cells from oxidative stress. It also plays a role in regulating immune responses.

5. **Zinc:** Zinc is involved in the development and function of immune cells and is necessary for proper immune system function. Zinc deficiency can impair immune function and increase susceptibility to infections.

6. **Selenium:** Selenium is an essential mineral that supports the production and function of immune cells. It also has antioxidant properties.

7. **Iron:** Iron is necessary for the production of hemoglobin, which carries oxygen to immune cells. Adequate iron levels are important for the proper function of immune cells.

8. **Copper:** Copper is involved in the development and maintenance of the immune system. It supports the function of white blood cells.

9. **Vitamin B6 (Pyridoxine):** Vitamin B6 is required for the production of antibodies and immune cell development. It also plays a role in reducing inflammation.

10. **Folate (Vitamin B9):** Folate is essential for the development and function of immune cells. It also supports antibody production.

11. **Vitamin B12:** Vitamin B12 is necessary for the production of red and white blood cells, including immune cells. A deficiency can weaken the immune system.

12. **Copper:** Copper is involved in the development and maintenance of the immune system and supports the function of white blood cells.

13. **Magnesium:** Magnesium plays a role in immune cell function and has anti-inflammatory properties.

14. **Sulfur:** Sulfur is involved in the production of antibodies and has anti-inflammatory properties.

15. **Iodine:** Iodine is essential for thyroid function, which in turn influences immune system regulation.

It is important to note that a balanced and varied diet is the best way to ensure you get an adequate intake of these vitamins and minerals. Whole foods like fruits, vegetables, lean proteins, nuts, seeds, and whole grains provide a wide range of nutrients that support overall health and immune function.

While dietary supplements can be helpful in cases of deficiency or for individuals with specific dietary restrictions, it is generally recommended to meet your nutrient needs through a well-rounded diet whenever possible. If you have concerns about your nutrient intake or immune health, consider consulting with a healthcare provider or registered dietitian for personalized guidance.

More home remedies no one has heard about.

Certainly, here are some lesser-known home remedies that you may not have heard about. Please keep in mind that while these remedies are generally considered safe, individual reactions may vary. If you have specific health concerns or conditions, it is a good idea to consult with a healthcare provider before trying any new home remedy.

1. **Oil Pulling:** Oil pulling is an ancient Ayurvedic practice that involves swishing a tablespoon of coconut oil or sesame oil in your mouth for about 15-20 minutes. It is believed to help improve oral health by reducing bacteria and promoting gum health.

2. **Blackstrap Molasses for Menstrual Cramps:** Blackstrap molasses, which is rich in iron and other minerals, is sometimes used as a natural remedy for alleviating menstrual cramps. Mixing a tablespoon in warm water or tea and drinking it during your period may help ease discomfort.

3. **Neti Pot for Sinus Congestion:** A neti pot is a small, teapot-like device used to flush out the sinuses with a saline solution. It can help relieve sinus congestion and improve breathing. Make sure to use sterile, distilled, or boiled water when using a neti pot.

4. **Baking Soda for Heartburn:** Baking soda, when mixed with water, can act as an antacid and help relieve heartburn and indigestion. Be cautious with this remedy, as excessive use of baking soda can lead to electrolyte imbalances.

5. **Duct Tape for Warts:** Applying a small piece of duct tape to a wart for several days may help remove it. This method is thought to work by irritating the skin and stimulating the immune system to fight the wart virus.

6. **Apple Cider Vinegar for Dandruff:** Apple cider vinegar is sometimes used as a natural remedy for dandruff. Mix it with water and apply it to your scalp, then rinse thoroughly. The acidity of the vinegar is believed to help balance the pH of the scalp.

7. **Raisins Soaked in Gin for Arthritis:** Some people soak golden raisins in gin and let them sit overnight. The raisins absorb some of the gin, and it is believed that consuming a small amount daily can help alleviate arthritis symptoms. However, this remedy is not scientifically proven and should be used with caution.

8. **Cherries for Gout:** Cherries, especially tart cherries, are believed to have anti-inflammatory properties that may help reduce the pain and inflammation associated with gout. Drinking cherry juice or eating cherries regularly may be beneficial.

9. **Epsom Salt Bath for Muscle Aches:** Adding Epsom salt (magnesium sulfate) to a warm bath is thought to help relax muscles and ease soreness. Magnesium may be absorbed through the skin.

10. **Clove Oil for Toothache:** Clove oil has natural numbing properties and can be applied topically to a painful tooth or gum area to provide temporary relief from toothache. Be sure to dilute it with a carrier oil to avoid irritation.

Remember that individual responses to these remedies can vary, and what works for one person may not work for another. If you have underlying health conditions or are taking medications, it is always a good idea to consult with a healthcare provider before trying any home remedy. Additionally, for serious or persistent health issues, seek professional medical advice and treatment.

More home remedies that cure illness and fight off germs and viruses.

While home remedies can help alleviate symptoms and support your immune system, they should not be seen as a substitute for medical treatment when dealing with serious illnesses or infections. However, here are some additional home remedies that may help boost your immune system and provide relief from common illnesses and minor infections:

1. **Garlic:** Garlic is known for its antimicrobial and immune-boosting properties. Consuming raw garlic or adding it to your meals may help fight off infections and reduce the severity and duration of colds.

2. **Honey and Lemon:** A mixture of honey and lemon in warm water can soothe a sore throat and provide relief from coughing. Honey also has natural antimicrobial properties.

3. **Ginger Tea:** Ginger has anti-inflammatory and immune- boosting properties. Ginger tea can help relieve nausea, soothe a sore throat, and reduce inflammation.

4. **Turmeric:** Turmeric contains curcumin, a compound with anti- inflammatory and antioxidant properties. It may help reduce inflammation and alleviate symptoms of arthritis, respiratory infections, and digestive issues.

5. **Salt Gargle:** Gargling with warm saltwater can help ease a sore throat, reduce inflammation, and kill bacteria. Dissolve half a teaspoon of salt in warm water and gargle several times a day.

6. **Probiotics:** Probiotic-rich foods like yogurt or kefir can support gut health, which is intricately linked to the immune system. Consuming these foods may help maintain a healthy balance of gut bacteria.

7. **Chicken Soup:** Chicken soup is a classic home remedy for colds and respiratory infections. It provides hydration, warmth, and essential nutrients that can help soothe symptoms.

8. **Eucalyptus Oil:** Inhaling steam with a few drops of eucalyptus oil can help relieve nasal congestion and ease breathing difficulties. Be cautious not to apply eucalyptus oil directly to the skin, as it can be irritating.

9. **Cinnamon and Honey:** A mixture of cinnamon and honey may help soothe a cough and boost the immune system. Mix a pinch of cinnamon with a teaspoon of honey and consume it a few times a day.

10. **Oregano Oil:** Oregano oil contains compounds with antimicrobial properties. A few drops of oregano oil diluted in a carrier oil can be applied topically for skin infections or used in a diffuser for respiratory issues.

11. **Astragalus Root:** Astragalus is an herb used in traditional Chinese medicine to support the immune system. It is available in various forms, including teas and supplements.

12. **Peppermint Tea:** Peppermint tea can help relieve indigestion, soothe an upset stomach, and provide relief from headaches and sinus congestion.

13. **Echinacea:** Echinacea is an herbal remedy that some people use to reduce the severity and duration of colds and upper respiratory infections. It is available in various forms, including teas and supplements.

14. **Warm Compress:** A warm compress or heating pad can help alleviate muscle aches, menstrual cramps, and joint pain.

It is important to remember that while these home remedies can provide relief from symptoms and support your immune system, they are not a substitute for professional medical advice and treatment, especially for serious illnesses or infections. If you have concerns about your health, consult with a healthcare provider for proper diagnosis and guidance.

Want to know the foods that boost the immune system?

Eating a balanced and nutrient-rich diet is one of the best ways to support and boost your immune system. A diet that includes a variety of foods can provide the vitamins, minerals, antioxidants, and other nutrients your immune system needs to function optimally. Here are some foods that are known for their immune-boosting properties:

1. **Citrus Fruits:** Citrus fruits like oranges, grapefruits, lemons, and limes are high in vitamin C, which is known to boost the production of white blood cells, key players in the immune system. Other fruits like strawberries, kiwi, and guava is also rich in vitamin C.

2. **Berries:** Berries, such as blueberries, strawberries, raspberries, and blackberries, are packed with antioxidants like flavonoids and vitamin C, which can help protect cells from oxidative stress.

3. **Garlic:** Garlic contains allicin, a compound known for its immune-boosting and antimicrobial properties. It is also a source of vitamins C and B6.

4. **Ginger:** Ginger has anti-inflammatory and antioxidant properties. It can help reduce inflammation, soothe sore throats, and alleviate nausea.

5. **Turmeric:** Turmeric contains curcumin, which has anti-inflammatory and antioxidant effects. It may help support immune function and reduce inflammation.

6. **Yogurt:** Yogurt and other fermented foods like kefir are rich in probiotics, which are beneficial bacteria that support gut health. A healthy gut is linked to a strong immune system.

7. **Spinach and Other Leafy Greens:** Leafy greens like spinach, kale, and Swiss chard are high in vitamins C and E, as well as other antioxidants and fiber that support overall health.

8. **Almonds:** Almonds are a useful source of vitamin E, which is a powerful antioxidant that helps maintain the integrity of cell membranes.

9. **Sunflower Seeds:** Sunflower seeds are rich in vitamin E, zinc, and selenium, all of which are important for immune function.

10. **Red Bell Peppers:** Red bell peppers are an excellent source of vitamin C and also provide beta carotene, which your body can convert into vitamin A, another immune-boosting nutrient.

11. **Poultry:** Chicken and turkey are rich in protein and contain nutrients like vitamin B6, which is important for immune function. Chicken soup, in particular, is a comfort food that can help soothe cold and flu symptoms.

12. **Shellfish:** Shellfish, such as crab, clams, and mussels, are high in zinc, a mineral that supports immune cell function.

13. **Mushrooms:** Certain mushrooms, like shiitake and maitake mushrooms, contain beta-glucans, compounds that have been shown to enhance immune function.

14. **Oats:** Oats and oatmeal are a source of beta-glucans, similar to those found in mushrooms, which may help boost immunity.

15. **Water:** Staying hydrated is essential for overall health, including immune function. Water helps flush toxins from the body and keeps your cells functioning optimally.

16. **Protein-Rich Foods:** Protein is important for the production of antibodies and immune cells. Include lean sources of protein like lean meat, poultry, fish, tofu, and legumes in your diet.

A well-balanced diet that incorporates a variety of these foods can provide your immune system with the nutrients it needs to function at its best. Additionally, maintaining a healthy lifestyle with regular exercise, adequate sleep, and stress management can further support a robust immune system.

The benefits of probiotics.

Probiotics are live microorganisms, often referred to as "good" or "friendly" bacteria, which provide a range of health benefits when consumed in adequate amounts. They are most commonly known for their positive impact on gut health, but their benefits extend to various other aspects of well-being. Here are some of the key benefits of probiotics:

1. **Improved Gut Health:** Probiotics help maintain a healthy balance of beneficial bacteria in the gut. They can support digestion, prevent the overgrowth of harmful bacteria, and promote regular bowel movements. Probiotics are particularly beneficial for individuals with conditions like irritable bowel syndrome (IBS), constipation, or diarrhea.

2. **Enhanced Immune Function:** A sizable portion of the immune system resides in the gut. Probiotics can help modulate the immune response and improve the body's ability to defend against infections. They may also reduce the severity and duration of colds and respiratory infections.

3. **Reduced Inflammation:** Certain probiotic strains have anti-inflammatory properties and can help mitigate chronic inflammation, which is linked to various health conditions, including inflammatory bowel disease (IBD), arthritis, and even some neurological disorders.

4. **Management of Gastrointestinal Conditions:** Probiotics can be effective in managing specific gastrointestinal conditions like inflammatory bowel disease (IBD), irritable bowel syndrome (IBS), and gastroenteritis (stomach flu).

5. **Prevention of Antibiotic-Related Diarrhea:** Taking probiotics during and after a course of antibiotics can help prevent.

antibiotic-associated diarrhea, which occurs when antibiotics disrupt the balance of gut bacteria.

6. **Support for Mental Health:** Emerging research suggests that the gut-brain connection, known as the gut-brain axis, may influence mental health. Probiotics may play a role in improving mood and reducing symptoms of anxiety and depression.

7. **Allergy Prevention:** Some studies suggest that probiotics, when taken during pregnancy or early childhood, may reduce the risk of allergies, including eczema and food allergies, in infants.

8. **Oral Health:** Probiotics can help maintain oral health by promoting a balanced oral microbiome, reducing the growth of harmful bacteria in the mouth, and preventing conditions like gingivitis and bad breath.

9. **Support for Women's Health:** Probiotics may help prevent and manage vaginal infections like yeast infections and bacterial vaginosis. They can also support overall urogenital health.

10. **Weight Management:** While more research is needed, some studies suggest that certain probiotics may help with weight loss and obesity management by influencing metabolism and appetite regulation.

11. **Lactose Digestion:** Probiotics containing lactase-producing strains can assist with lactose digestion in individuals with lactose intolerance.

12. **Enhanced Nutrient Absorption:** Probiotics can improve the absorption of certain nutrients, such as calcium, magnesium, and certain B vitamins.

It is important to note that the benefits of probiotics can vary depending on the specific strains and dosages used. Probiotics are available in various forms, including supplements and fermented foods like yogurt, kefir, sauerkraut, and kimchi. If you are considering adding probiotics to your diet or taking them as supplements, it is a good idea to consult with a healthcare provider or registered dietitian to ensure you choose the right strains and dosages for your specific health goals and needs. Additionally, individual responses to probiotics can vary, so it may take some trial and error to find the most beneficial strains for you.

Here are the benefits of probiotics for weight loss.

The relationship between probiotics and weight loss is an area of ongoing research, and while there is some evidence to suggest a potential connection, it is important to approach the topic with caution. Probiotics are primarily known for their role in gut health, but their effects on weight management are complex and can vary depending on several factors. Here are some of the ways probiotics may be associated with weight management:

1. **Improved Gut Health:** Probiotics can help maintain a healthy balance of gut bacteria, which is important for digestion and

nutrient absorption. An imbalanced gut microbiome has been linked to weight gain and obesity.

2. **Influence on Metabolism:** Some research suggests that certain probiotic strains may influence metabolism, including the way the body processes and stores fat. This can potentially have an impact on weight management.

3. **Appetite Regulation:** Probiotics may affect appetite-regulating hormones and signals in the gut, which can influence food intake and cravings.

4. **Reduced Inflammation:** Chronic inflammation is associated with obesity, and some probiotics have anti-inflammatory properties. Reducing inflammation may help with weight management.

5. **Improved Insulin Sensitivity:** Certain probiotics may help improve insulin sensitivity, which can have a positive effect on blood sugar control and weight management.

6. **Reduced Fat Absorption:** Some probiotic strains may inhibit the absorption of dietary fat in the intestines, potentially leading to a lower calorie intake.

7. **Support for Healthy Eating Habits:** Probiotics may influence food choices and preferences by affecting the gut-brain axis. A balanced gut microbiome can potentially reduce cravings for unhealthy foods.

It is important to note that the effects of probiotics on weight are modest, and they should not be seen as a magic solution for weight loss. Individual responses to probiotics can vary widely, and their impact on weight management is influenced by several factors, including genetics, diet, lifestyle, and the specific strains and doses used.

If you are interested in incorporating probiotics into your weight management plan, here are some tips:

1. **Choose the Right Strains:** Certain strains of probiotics, such as Lactobacillus gassier and Bifidobacterium breve, have been studied for their potential role in weight management. Look for supplements that contain these strains if you are considering probiotic supplementation.

2. **Diet and Lifestyle:** Probiotics are most effective when combined with a healthy diet and regular physical activity. They are not a substitute for a balanced lifestyle.

3. **Consult a Healthcare Provider:** Before starting any new supplement, especially for weight management, it is advisable to consult with a healthcare provider or registered dietitian. They can provide guidance based on your individual health needs and goals.

In summary, while there is some evidence to suggest that probiotics may have a role in supporting weight management, more research is needed to fully understand their mechanisms and effectiveness. Probiotics can be a valuable addition to a healthy lifestyle but should not be relied upon as the sole solution for weight loss.

What are fermented foods with probiotics?

Fermented foods are a rich source of probiotics, which are beneficial live bacteria that can support gut health and overall well-being. Including these foods in your diet can help maintain a healthy balance of gut bacteria. Here are some popular fermented foods that are rich in probiotics:

1. **Yogurt:** Yogurt is one of the most well-known probiotic-rich foods. Look for yogurt with "live and active cultures" on the label to ensure it contains probiotics. Greek yogurt and other plain, unsweetened yogurts tend to have higher probiotic content.

2. **Kefir:** Kefir is a fermented milk drink that is similar to yogurt but has a thinner consistency. It is made by fermenting milk with kefir grains, which are a combination of bacteria and yeast.

3. **Sauerkraut:** Sauerkraut is fermented cabbage and is a staple in many traditional diets. It is rich in probiotics and has a tangy flavor.

4. **Kimchi:** Kimchi is a spicy fermented cabbage dish that is a staple in Korean cuisine. It is made with a variety of seasonings and vegetables, and it is a potent source of probiotics.

5. **Miso:** Miso is a traditional Japanese seasoning made by fermenting soybeans or other legumes with salt and a type of fungus called koji. It is commonly used to make soup and adds a rich, umami flavor.

6. **Tempeh:** Tempeh is a fermented soybean product that originated in Indonesia. It has a nutty flavor and a firm texture. It is a source of both probiotics and plant-based protein.

7. **Pickles (fermented in brine):** Traditional pickles that are fermented in brine rather than made with vinegar contain probiotics. Look for pickles that are labeled as "naturally fermented" or "fermented in brine."

8. **Natto:** Natto is a Japanese dish made from fermented soybeans. It has a distinctive taste and a sticky texture. Natto is a source of probiotics and vitamin K2.

9. **Kombucha:** Kombucha is a fermented tea beverage that is becoming increasingly popular. It is made by fermenting sweet tea with a SCOBY (symbiotic culture of bacteria and yeast). Kombucha can contain a variety of probiotic strains.

10. **Traditional Buttermilk:** Traditional buttermilk is the liquid left behind after churning butter. It is cultured and often used in baking and cooking.

11. **Lassi:** Lassi is a traditional Indian yogurt-based drink that can be flavored with fruit or spices. It is a source of probiotics and is often consumed as a refreshing beverage.

When incorporating fermented foods into your diet for their probiotic benefits, be sure to choose options that are minimally processed and free of additives, as processing can destroy beneficial bacteria.

Additionally, it is important to consume a variety of fermented foods to expose your gut to different strains of probiotics for maximum benefit.

As with any dietary change, if you have specific dietary restrictions or health concerns, consult with a healthcare provider or register.

dietitian to ensure that fermented foods are appropriate for your individual needs and preferences.

Best home remedy to promote anemic (low iron)

Anemia, especially iron-deficiency anemia, is a condition where your body lacks enough red blood cells or hemoglobin to carry sufficient oxygen to your body's tissues. While home remedies can help improve your iron status to some extent, it is important to remember that they are not a replacement for medical treatment. If you suspect you have anemia, it is crucial to consult with a healthcare provider for proper diagnosis and guidance. In addition to any treatment or supplements recommended by your healthcare provider, you can consider these home remedies to support your iron levels:

1. *DIETARY CHANGES:*

   - **Iron-Rich Foods:** Include iron-rich foods in your diet, such as lean meats, poultry, fish, beans, lentils, tofu, spinach, fortified cereals, and dried fruits like raisins and apricots. These foods provide heme and non-heme iron, which your body can absorb.
   - **Vitamin C:** Consume foods rich in vitamin C (ascorbic acid), such as citrus fruits, strawberries, kiwi, and bell peppers. Vitamin C enhances the absorption of non- heme iron from plant-based sources when consumed together.

2. *COOKING TECHNIQUES:*

- **Cast-Iron Cookware:** Cooking with cast-iron pans can increase the iron content of your meals, especially if you cook acidic foods like tomatoes in them.

3. *HERBAL REMEDIES:*

- **Nettle Tea:** Nettle tea is sometimes recommended as a natural remedy for anemia. It contains iron and other nutrients that can support iron levels. Consult with a healthcare provider before adding herbal remedies to your diet, especially if you are pregnant, nursing, or taking medications.

4. *AVOID IRON INHIBITORS'*

- o **Tea and Coffee:** Reduce your consumption of tea and coffee, particularly around mealtimes. These beverages contain compounds that can inhibit iron absorption.

- **Limit Calcium Supplements:** If you take calcium supplements, avoid taking them with iron-rich meals, as calcium can interfere with iron absorption.

- *HEALTHY LIFESTYLE:*

- o **Moderate Exercise:** Engage in regular, moderate exercise to promote overall health and well-being. Consult with your healthcare provider before starting a new exercise routine.

- **Stay Hydrated:** Ensure that you drink enough water daily to support overall health and bodily functions.

- **Supplements:** If recommended by your healthcare provider, you may need iron supplements. Iron supplements should be taken under the guidance of a healthcare professional, as excessive iron intake can have adverse effects.

5. **Monitor Progress:** Periodically check your iron levels through blood tests to track your progress and adjust your approach if needed.

It is crucial to consult with a healthcare provider to determine the cause of your anemia, as the appropriate treatment can vary depending on the underlying issue. Iron supplements may be necessary in cases of severe deficiency or when dietary changes alone are insufficient.

Remember that dietary changes and home remedies take time to impact iron levels, so be patient and consistent with your efforts. If you experience symptoms of anemia, such as fatigue, weakness, pale skin, or shortness of breath, consult with a healthcare provider promptly for a proper evaluation and personalized treatment plan.

I recommend these for iron-rich recipes.

Certainly! Here are some iron-rich recipes that incorporate a variety of foods to help boost your iron intake. Keep in mind that the iron content of these recipes can vary based on portion sizes and ingredient choices, so you may want to adjust them to suit your dietary preferences and nutritional needs.

1. *SPINACH AND CHICKPEA SALAD:*

   - Ingredients:

     - Fresh spinach leaves

     - Cooked chickpeas

     - Cherry tomatoes

     - Red onion (sliced)

     - Feta cheese (optional)

     - Olive oil and balsamic vinegar dressing

     - Sunflower seeds (for added crunch and iron)

   - Instructions:

     - Toss all the ingredients together in a bowl and drizzle with dressing.

2. *LENTIL AND VEGETABLE CURRY:*

   - Ingredients:

     - Red or green lentils

     - Mixed vegetables (e.g., carrots, bell peppers, zucchini)
     - Coconut milk

- Curry spices (turmeric, cumin, coriander, ginger)

- Onion and garlic

- Serve with brown rice or whole-grain naan.

- Instructions:

  - Sauté onion and garlic in a pot, then add lentils, vegetables, coconut milk, and spices.
  - Simmer until the lentils and vegetables are tender and serve over rice or with naan.

3. *BEEF AND BROCCOLI STIR-FRY:*

- Ingredients:

  - Lean beef strips

  - Broccoli florets

  - Soy sauce

  - Garlic and ginger (minced)

  - Brown rice or quinoa

- Instructions:

  - Stir-fry beef in a pan with garlic and ginger until cooked.
  - Add broccoli and soy sauce, and stir-fry until tender.
  - Serve over cooked brown rice or quinoa.

4. *CHICKPEA AND SPINACH CURRY:*

- Ingredients:

  - Chickpeas (canned or cooked)

  - Fresh spinach leaves

  - Coconut milk

  - Curry spices (turmeric, cumin, garam masala)

  - Onion and garlic

  - Serve with brown rice or whole-grain flatbread.

- Instructions:

  - Sauté onion and garlic, then add chickpeas, spinach, coconut milk, and spices.
  - Simmer until spinach is wilted and serve over rice or with flatbread.

5. *SALMON AND QUINOA BOWL:*

- Ingredients:

  - Grilled or baked salmon

  - Cooked quinoa

  - Steamed broccoli.

  - Sliced avocado

  - Lemon dill sauce (made with yogurt, lemon juice, and dill)

- Instructions:

- Assemble the ingredients in a bowl and drizzle with lemon dill sauce.

6. *IRON-RICH SMOOTHIE:*

- Ingredients:

  - Spinach or kale

  - Frozen berries

  - Banana

  - Greek yogurt or almond milk

  - Chia seeds (for added iron and fiber)

- Instructions:

  - Blend all the ingredients until smooth and enjoy as a nutritious breakfast or snack.

These recipes incorporate a variety of iron-rich foods, including leafy greens, legumes, lean meats, and whole grains. Remember to balance your iron intake with foods high in vitamin C, which can enhance iron absorption, and avoid consuming calcium-rich foods or supplements with iron-rich meals, as calcium can inhibit iron absorption.

Best sources of Magnesium

Magnesium is an essential mineral that plays a crucial role in various bodily functions, including muscle and nerve function, blood glucose control, and bone health. It is important to ensure you are getting an adequate intake of magnesium through your diet. Here are some of the best dietary sources of magnesium:

1. *NUTS AND SEEDS:*

- Almonds
- Cashews
    - Pumpkin seeds
    - Sunflower seeds

2. *LEGUMES:*

    - Black beans
    - Chickpeas (garbanzo beans)
    - Lentils
    - Peas

3. *WHOLE GRAINS:*

   - Brown rice

   - Oats

   - Quinoa

   - Whole wheat pasta

4. *LEAFY GREENS:*

   - Spinach

   - Swiss chard

   - Kale

   - Collard greens

5. *FISH:*

   - Salmon

   - Mackerel

   - Halibut

6. **Avocado:** Avocado is a nutrient-rich fruit that contains magnesium along with healthy fats and fiber.

7. **Dark Chocolate:** High-quality dark chocolate with a cocoa content of 70% or more is a source of magnesium.

8. **Bananas:** Bananas are a useful source of magnesium and are also rich in potassium.

9. **Yogurt:** Plain yogurt, particularly Greek yogurt, contains magnesium, along with beneficial probiotics and protein.

10. **Tofu:** Tofu is a soy-based product that provides magnesium and is an excellent source of plant-based protein.
11. **Figs:** Dried figs are a concentrated source of magnesium, fiber, and natural sugars.
12. **Seaweed:** Some types of seaweed, like dried nori sheets used in sushi, contain magnesium.
13. **Blackstrap Molasses:** Blackstrap molasses is a byproduct of sugar production and is rich in magnesium and other minerals.
14. **Pumpkin:** Pumpkin, whether fresh or canned, is a source of magnesium and other nutrients.
15. **Whole-Grain Bread:** Whole-grain bread made from whole wheat flour can contribute to your magnesium intake.

It is important to maintain a balanced diet that includes a variety of these magnesium-rich foods to meet your daily magnesium needs. The recommended dietary allowance (RDA) for magnesium varies by age and sex but typically ranges from 310 to 420 milligrams per day for most adults. However, individual magnesium requirements may vary based on factors such as age, sex, activity level, and overall health.

If you have specific concerns about your magnesium intake or are considering magnesium supplements, it is a good idea to consult with a healthcare provider or registered dietitian for personalized guidance. They can help you figure out if supplementation is necessary and recommend a suitable dosage based on your individual needs.

What are the benefits of magnesium?

Magnesium is an essential mineral that plays a crucial role in numerous bodily functions. It takes part in over three hundred biochemical reactions in the body, making it vital for overall health and well-being. Here are some of the key benefits and roles of magnesium in the body:

1. **Muscle Function:** Magnesium is essential for muscle contraction and relaxation. It helps regulate muscle contractions and prevents muscle cramps and spasms.

2. **Nerve Function:** Magnesium is important for nerve transmission and the regulation of neurotransmitters, which are chemical messengers in the brain.

3. **Energy Production:** Magnesium is a co-factor for enzymes involved in energy metabolism. It helps convert food into energy and supports overall vitality.

4. **Heart Health:** Magnesium plays a role in keeping a regular heartbeat and supporting cardiovascular health. It helps relax blood vessels, which can help lower blood pressure.

5. **Bone Health:** About 60-70% of the body's magnesium is stored in the bones, where it contributes to bone density and helps prevent osteoporosis.

6. **Blood Sugar Regulation:** Magnesium helps regulate blood sugar levels by influencing insulin sensitivity. Adequate magnesium intake may reduce the risk of type 2 diabetes.

7. **Immune System Support:** Magnesium supports the immune system by promoting the production and function of immune cells.

8. **Stress Management:** Magnesium may help reduce stress and anxiety by regulating the release of stress hormones and promoting relaxation.

9. **Mood Enhancement:** Adequate magnesium levels are associated with improved mood and a reduced risk of depression.

10. **Digestive Health:** Magnesium helps maintain proper muscle function in the digestive tract, promoting regular bowel movements and preventing constipation.

11. **Blood Pressure Regulation:** Magnesium can help lower blood pressure by relaxing blood vessels and improving blood flow.

12. **Headache and Migraine Relief:** Some people find that magnesium supplements or magnesium-rich foods can reduce the frequency and severity of headaches and migraines.

13. **PMS Symptom Relief:** Magnesium may help alleviate symptoms of premenstrual syndrome (PMS), such as bloating and mood swings.

14. **Anti-Inflammatory Effects:** Magnesium has anti-inflammatory properties that may help reduce chronic inflammation in the body, which is linked to various health conditions.

15. **Better Sleep:** Magnesium can support healthy sleep patterns by promoting relaxation and reducing insomnia and restless leg syndrome.

While magnesium is readily available in a variety of foods, some individuals may have a higher risk of magnesium deficiency, including those with certain medical conditions, digestive disorders, or those taking medications that interfere with magnesium absorption. In such cases, magnesium supplements may be recommended under the guidance of a healthcare provider.

It is important to maintain a balanced diet that includes magnesium-rich foods to support your overall health. If you suspect you have a magnesium deficiency or have specific health concerns, consult with a healthcare provider for proper evaluation and guidance. Taking excessive magnesium supplements can lead to adverse effects, so it is essential to discuss supplementation with a healthcare professional.

What are the symptoms of magnesium deficiency?

Magnesium deficiency, also known as hypomagnesemia, can manifest with a range of symptoms, and its signs can vary from mild to severe. Since magnesium is involved in numerous bodily functions, a deficiency can affect various systems in the body. Common symptoms of magnesium deficiency include:

1. **Muscle Cramps and Spasms:** Magnesium plays a vital role in muscle contraction and relaxation. Deficiency can lead to muscle cramps, spasms, and muscle weakness.
2. **Fatigue and Weakness:** Low magnesium levels can contribute to overall fatigue, weakness, and a lack of energy.
3. **Nausea and Vomiting:** Some individuals with magnesium deficiency may experience nausea and vomiting.

4. **Loss of Appetite:** A diminished appetite or changes in taste can occur with magnesium deficiency.

5. **Numbness and Tingling:** Magnesium deficiency may lead to tingling or numbness, particularly in the extremities.

6. **Tremors:** Some people with low magnesium levels may experience tremors or shakiness.

7. **Personality Changes:** Magnesium plays a role in mood regulation, and deficiency can contribute to mood changes, including increased irritability and anxiety.

8. **Heart Palpitations:** Magnesium is involved in maintaining a regular heartbeat. Deficiency can lead to irregular heart rhythms or palpitations.

9. **High Blood Pressure:** Low magnesium levels can be associated with elevated blood pressure.

10. **Constipation:** Magnesium helps regulate muscle function in the digestive tract. A deficiency can lead to constipation.

11. **Muscle Weakness:** Severe magnesium deficiency can cause muscle weakness, which may impair mobility.

12. **Seizures:** In extreme cases, magnesium deficiency can lead to seizures, though this is relatively rare.

It is important to note that magnesium deficiency may go unrecognized or be mistaken for other conditions because its symptoms can overlap with those of various health issues. If you suspect you have a magnesium deficiency or experience persistent symptoms, consult with a healthcare provider for proper evaluation and testing. Blood tests can help determine your magnesium levels and guide treatment if deficiency is confirmed.

Magnesium deficiency can result from inadequate dietary intake, digestive disorders that interfere with absorption, certain medications, alcohol abuse, or medical conditions that lead to increased magnesium loss (e.g., kidney disorders). Treatment typically involves dietary changes, magnesium supplements, or addressing the underlying cause, depending on the severity of the deficiency.

Here is some home remedies that help with infections.

Home remedies can be helpful in managing mild infections and relieving symptoms. However, it is important to note that for serious or persistent infections, consulting with a healthcare professional is crucial, as antibiotics or other medical treatments may be necessary. Here are some home remedies that may provide relief for mild infections:

1. **Saltwater Gargle:** A warm saltwater gargle can help soothe a sore throat and reduce inflammation. Dissolve half a teaspoon of salt in a glass of warm water and gargle with it several times a day.

2. **Honey:** Honey has natural antibacterial properties and can help soothe a sore throat and cough. Mix a teaspoon of honey in warm water or herbal tea and drink it.

3. **Garlic:** Garlic contains compounds with antimicrobial properties. Eating raw garlic or adding it to your meals may help fight infections. If you do not like the taste of raw garlic, you can also take garlic supplements (with the guidance of a healthcare provider).

4. **Ginger:** Ginger has anti-inflammatory and antimicrobial properties. You can make ginger tea by steeping fresh ginger slices in hot water. Adding honey and lemon can enhance its soothing effects.

5. **Turmeric:** Turmeric contains curcumin, a compound known for its anti-inflammatory and antibacterial properties. You can add turmeric to soups, stews, or warm milk for consumption.

6. **Steam Inhalation:** Inhaling steam from a bowl of hot water can help relieve congestion and ease sinus and respiratory infections. You can add a few drops of essential oils like eucalyptus or peppermint for added relief.

7. **Probiotics:** Consuming foods rich in probiotics (e.g., yogurt with live cultures) or taking probiotic supplements may help support your immune system and maintain a healthy gut microbiome.

8. **Tea Tree Oil:** Tea tree oil has antimicrobial properties and can be diluted with a carrier oil (such as coconut oil) and applied topically to skin infections like acne or fungal infections.

9. **Echinacea:** Echinacea is an herb that is often used to boost the immune system. Echinacea supplements or herbal teas may

help reduce the duration and severity of colds and respiratory infections.

10. **Warm Compress:** Applying a warm compress to infected areas (e.g., a warm, damp cloth on a skin boil) can help promote drainage and relieve discomfort.
11. **Rest and Hydration:** Adequate rest and hydration are essential for your body to fight off infections. Make sure you get plenty of sleep and drink fluids like water, herbal teas, and clear broths.
12. **Maintain Good Hygiene:** Proper handwashing, regular bathing, and keeping the affected area clean are essential for preventing the spread of infections.

It is important to remember that while home remedies can provide relief from mild infections and support your body's natural healing processes, they are not a substitute for professional medical advice and treatment. If you have a severe infection, persistent symptoms, or underlying health conditions, consult with a healthcare provider for proper evaluation and treatment. Additionally, if you are allergic to any ingredients or experience adverse reactions to home remedies, discontinue use and seek medical advice.

Natural remedies for sore throat?

Sore throats are a common ailment, often caused by viral infections like the common cold or the flu. While home remedies can help alleviate the discomfort associated with a sore throat, it is essential to consult a healthcare provider if your symptoms persist or worsen. Here are some natural remedies to soothe a sore throat:

1. **Warm Saltwater Gargle:** Gargling with warm saltwater can help reduce throat inflammation and relieve pain. Dissolve half a teaspoon of salt in a glass of warm water and gargle for about 30 seconds before spitting it out. Repeat several times a day.

2. **Honey and Warm Water:** Honey has natural antibacterial properties and can soothe a sore throat. Mix a teaspoon of honey into a cup of warm water or herbal tea and sip it slowly.

3. **Herbal Teas:** Herbal teas like chamomile, ginger, and peppermint can provide relief. These teas are often soothing and can help ease throat discomfort. Add honey for extra comfort.

4. **Lemon Water:** Lemon juice can help break up mucus and provide vitamin C, which may support your immune system. Mix the juice of half a lemon in a cup of warm water and add honey to taste.

5. **Apple Cider Vinegar:** Mix a teaspoon of apple cider vinegar with a cup of warm water. Gargle with this solution several times a day. The acidity of the vinegar can help kill bacteria and soothe your throat.

6. **Slippery Elm:** Slippery elm lozenges or teas are known for their throat-soothing properties. The mucilage in slippery elm can coat and protect the throat.

7. **Humidifier:** Use a humidifier in your room to add moisture to the air. Dry air can worsen throat irritation, and a humidifier can help keep your throat comfortable, especially during the night.

8. **Saltwater Nasal Rinse:** If your sore throat is due to postnasal drip, a saline nasal rinse can help clear mucus and reduce irritation in the throat.

9. **Popsicles or Ice Chips:** Cold treats like popsicles or ice chips can temporarily numb the throat and provide relief.

10. **Rest and Hydration:** Adequate rest and hydration are crucial for your body to recover from infections. Make sure to drink plenty of fluids to stay hydrated and support your immune system.

11. **Avoid Irritants:** Avoid smoking and exposure to secondhand smoke, as well as irritants like strong odors or pollutants that can worsen throat irritation.

12. **Cinnamon and Ginger Tea:** Cinnamon and ginger have anti-inflammatory and soothing properties. Brew tea by steeping cinnamon sticks and ginger slices in hot water. Add honey and lemon for flavor and relief.

13. **Marshmallow Root Tea:** Marshmallow root is known for its mucilaginous properties, which can help soothe a sore throat. Make tea by steeping marshmallow root in hot water.

Remember that while these natural remedies can provide relief from sore throat symptoms, they are not a substitute for medical evaluation and treatment, especially if you have a severe sore throat, difficulty swallowing, a high fever, or if your symptoms persist for more than a few days. Consult with a healthcare provider if you are concerned about your sore throat or if you experience any alarming symptoms.

5. **Preparation Methods:** Herbal remedies can be prepared in various forms, such as teas, tinctures (liquid extracts), capsules, ointments, and salves. The chosen preparation method often depends on the plant and the intended use.

6. **Safety and Quality:** The safety and efficacy of herbal remedies can vary widely. It is essential to source high-quality herbs and follow recommended dosages. Consultation with a qualified herbalist or healthcare provider is advisable, especially if you have underlying health conditions or are taking medications.

7. **Scientific Research:** Some herbal remedies have been studied extensively through scientific research, supplying evidence for their efficacy and safety. Others are based more on traditional knowledge and anecdotal evidence.

8. **Regulation:** The regulation of herbal remedies varies by country. In some regions, herbal products are subject to specific regulations and quality standards. In others, they may be available as dietary supplements with less oversight.

9. **Complementary Medicine:** Herbal medicine is often used in conjunction with conventional medical treatments as complementary therapy. It is important to inform your healthcare provider about any herbal remedies you are using, as they can interact with medications or other treatments.

10. **Individualized Treatment:** Herbalists often tailor remedies to the individual, considering factors like age, gender, overall health, and specific symptoms. This personalized approach is a hallmark of herbal medicine.

11. **Cautions and Contraindications:** Some herbs can have side effects or interactions with medications. Pregnant and nursing

Individuals, as well as those with certain medical conditions, should exercise caution when using herbal remedies.

Popular herbs used in herbal medicine include echinacea, ginseng, chamomile, lavender, peppermint, valerian, and many others. It is important to note that the effectiveness of herbal remedies can vary from person to person, and not all herbs are suitable for every individual or condition.

If you are considering using herbal remedies for a specific health concern, it is advisable to consult with a qualified herbalist, naturopathic doctor, or healthcare provider who can provide guidance and ensure safe and effective use. Additionally, be sure to inform your healthcare provider about any herbal remedies you are using to avoid potential interactions with medications or medical treatments.

Want to know more common herbal remedies?

Common herbal remedies have been used for generations to address a variety of health concerns. Here are some well-known herbal remedies, along with the health issues they are often used to treat or manage:

1. **Echinacea:** Echinacea is often used to support the immune system and may help reduce the severity and duration of colds and upper respiratory infections.

2. **Ginseng:** Ginseng, including American ginseng and Asian ginseng, is used for its potential to boost energy, improve cognitive function, and support overall vitality.

3. **Chamomile:** Chamomile is known for its calming properties and is used to relieve stress, anxiety, and insomnia. It is also used to soothe digestive discomfort.

4. **Peppermint:** Peppermint is used to alleviate digestive issues, including indigestion, bloating, and gas. It is also known for its soothing effects on headaches.

5. **Valerian:** Valerian root is a natural remedy for insomnia and sleep disorders. It is used for its sedative properties to promote better sleep.

6. **Lavender:** Lavender is used for its calming and relaxation-inducing effects. It is often used in aromatherapy and as an essential oil for stress relief.

7. **St. John's Wort:** St. John's Wort is used as a natural remedy for mild to moderate depression and mood disorders. It may also help with anxiety.

8. **Turmeric:** Turmeric contains curcumin, a compound with anti-inflammatory and antioxidant properties. It is used for its potential to reduce inflammation and alleviate pain, especially in conditions like arthritis.

9. **Ginger:** Ginger is known for its digestive benefits and is often used to relieve nausea, motion sickness, and indigestion. It also has anti-inflammatory properties.

10. **Milk Thistle:** Milk thistle is used to support liver health and detoxification. It may be used in cases of liver damage or conditions like fatty liver disease.

11. **Saw Palmetto:** Saw palmetto is commonly used to alleviate symptoms of an enlarged prostate (benign prostatic hyperplasia or BPH) and may help with urinary tract issues.

12. **Elderberry:** Elderberry is known for its potential to boost the immune system and reduce the severity and duration of cold and flu symptoms.

13. **Garlic:** Garlic is used for its immune-boosting properties and potential to lower blood pressure and cholesterol levels. It is also known for its antimicrobial effects.

14. **Arnica:** Arnica is applied topically in the form of creams or gels and is used for its potential to reduce pain and inflammation associated with bruises, sprains, and muscle soreness.

15. **Ginkgo Biloba:** Ginkgo biloba is used to support cognitive function and may improve memory and concentration. It is often used in cases of age-related cognitive decline.

It is important to note that while these herbal remedies have been used for various health concerns, their effectiveness can vary from person to person. Additionally, some herbs may interact with medications or have contraindications, so it is crucial to consult with a qualified herbalist or healthcare provider before using herbal remedies, especially if you have underlying health conditions or are taking medications. Individualized guidance can help ensure safe and effective use of herbal remedies.

Here is more about ginger benefits.

Ginger is a versatile and widely used spice that has been treasured for its culinary and medicinal properties for centuries. It is derived from the rhizome (underground stem) of the Zingiber officinale plant and is known for its distinctive flavor and aroma. Ginger offers a range of health benefits due to its rich composition of bioactive compounds, including gingerol, which is the primary bioactive compound responsible for many of its therapeutic effects. Here are some key benefits and uses of ginger:

1. **Digestive Health:** Ginger has long been used to relieve various digestive issues, including indigestion, bloating, and gas. It can help stimulate the digestive tract, reduce nausea, and alleviate motion sickness.

2. **Nausea and Morning Sickness:** Ginger is effective in reducing nausea and vomiting, making it a popular remedy for morning sickness during pregnancy and nausea associated with chemotherapy and surgery.

3. **Anti-Inflammatory Properties:** Ginger has natural anti-inflammatory properties, and its regular consumption may help reduce inflammation in the body. This can be particularly beneficial for individuals with osteoarthritis or inflammatory conditions.

4. **Pain Relief:** Ginger has analgesic properties and may help reduce pain associated with conditions like arthritis, muscle soreness, and menstrual cramps.

5. **Immune System Support:** Ginger contains antioxidants that support the immune system and may help reduce the risk of infections. It can be especially beneficial during cold and flu season.

6. **Lowering Blood Sugar:** Some studies suggest that ginger may help improve insulin sensitivity and lower blood sugar levels in individuals with type 2 diabetes.

7. **Cardiovascular Health:** Ginger may have a positive impact on heart health by reducing blood pressure and cholesterol levels. It can also help reduce the risk of blood clot formation.

8. **Cognitive Function:** Emerging research suggests that ginger may have potential cognitive benefits, including improving memory and cognitive function.

9. **Menstrual Pain Relief:** Ginger may help alleviate menstrual pain and discomfort when consumed regularly during the menstrual cycle.

10. **Weight Management:** Some studies indicate that ginger may support weight management by increasing feelings of fullness and promoting fat burning.

11. **Antimicrobial Effects:** Ginger exhibits antimicrobial properties that may help combat bacterial and fungal infections.

12. **Cancer Prevention:** Preliminary research suggests that ginger may have potential cancer-fighting properties, but further studies are needed to confirm these effects.

13. **Skin Health:** Ginger's anti-inflammatory and antioxidant properties may contribute to improved skin health, helping to reduce skin aging and acne.

Ginger can be consumed in various forms, including fresh ginger root, ginger tea, ginger supplements, and as an ingredient in cooking and baking. It can be used to flavor both sweet and savory dishes, and ginger tea is a popular beverage for its soothing and digestive benefits.

While ginger is generally considered safe when consumed in moderate amounts, excessive intake may lead to digestive discomfort or other side effects in some individuals. If you have specific health concerns or are considering ginger supplements, it is advisable to consult with a healthcare provider for personalized guidance, especially if you are pregnant, nursing, or taking medications.

Want to know more about turmeric's benefits.

Turmeric, known scientifically as Curcuma longa, is a bright yellow spice commonly used in Indian and Southeast Asian cuisine. It has been used for thousands of years in traditional medicine due to its remarkable health benefits. The active compound in turmeric responsible for many of its therapeutic effects is curcumin. Here are some of the key benefits and uses of turmeric:

1. **Anti-Inflammatory Properties:** Curcumin is a powerful anti-inflammatory agent that helps reduce chronic inflammation in the body. Chronic inflammation is linked to many chronic diseases, including heart disease, cancer, and arthritis.

2. **Antioxidant Activity:** Turmeric contains antioxidants that neutralize harmful free radicals, helping protect cells from oxidative damage. This may contribute to its anti-aging and disease-fighting properties.

3. **Pain Relief:** Due to its anti-inflammatory properties, turmeric can help alleviate pain, making it useful for conditions like arthritis, joint pain, and muscle soreness.

4. **Joint Health:** Turmeric may improve symptoms of osteoarthritis and rheumatoid arthritis, thanks to its anti-inflammatory and pain-relieving effects.

5. **Digestive Health:** Turmeric can aid digestion by stimulating the gallbladder to produce bile, which helps break down fats. It may also alleviate symptoms of indigestion and bloating.

6. **Heart Health:** Some studies suggest that curcumin may improve heart health by improving endothelial function, reducing inflammation, and reducing the risk factors associated with heart disease.

7. **Brain Health:** Curcumin has shown promise in supporting brain health by promoting the production of brain-derived neurotrophic factor (BDNF), a growth hormone that functions in the brain. It may help delay or even reverse brain diseases and age-related decreases in brain function.

8. **Cancer Prevention:** Curcumin has anti-cancer properties and may help prevent and treat certain types of cancer. It inhibits the growth of cancer cells and suppresses the spread of tumors.

9. **Depression and Anxiety:** Some research suggests that curcumin may have a positive impact on mood disorders like depression.

and anxiety by increasing brain levels of serotonin and dopamine.

10. **Skin Health:** Turmeric is used in skincare for its anti-inflammatory and antioxidant properties. It may help reduce acne, promote wound healing, and improve the overall appearance of the skin.

11. **Immune Support:** Turmeric's immune-boosting properties may help the body defend against infections and support overall immune function.

12. **Liver Health:** Turmeric supports liver function by aiding in the detoxification process. It may help protect the liver from damage caused by toxins and alcohol.

13. **Weight Management:** Curcumin may assist in weight management by regulating metabolism and reducing fat tissue inflammation.

14. **Diabetes Management:** Some studies suggest that curcumin may improve insulin sensitivity and help lower blood sugar levels in individuals with type 2 diabetes.

Turmeric can be incorporated into the diet by adding it to curries, soups, stews, and rice dishes. Turmeric supplements containing curcumin are also available and can provide a more concentrated source of the active compound. However, it is important to note that curcumin is not well-absorbed on its own, so black pepper, which contains peperino, is often added to enhance absorption.

While turmeric is generally considered safe when used in cooking, excessive consumption of curcumin supplements may lead to digestive discomfort or interact with certain medications. If you have specific health concerns or are considering turmeric supplements, it is.

advisable to consult with a healthcare provider for personalized guidance.

Here are the benefits of turmeric.

Turmeric, a bright yellow spice commonly used in cooking and traditional medicine, offers a wide range of health benefits primarily due to its active compound, curcumin. Here are some of the key benefits of turmeric:

1. **Anti-Inflammatory Properties:** Curcumin, the primary bioactive compound in turmeric, has potent anti-inflammatory effects. It can help reduce chronic inflammation, which is associated with many chronic diseases, including heart disease, cancer, and arthritis.

2. **Antioxidant Activity:** Turmeric contains antioxidants that neutralize harmful free radicals, protecting cells and tissues from oxidative damage. This may contribute to its anti-aging and disease-fighting properties.

3. **Pain Relief:** Curcumin's anti-inflammatory properties can help alleviate pain, making it useful for conditions like osteoarthritis, rheumatoid arthritis, and muscle soreness.

4. **Joint Health:** Turmeric may improve joint health by reducing inflammation and pain associated with arthritis. It may also support overall joint function.

5. **Digestive Health:** Turmeric can aid digestion by stimulating the gallbladder to produce bile, which aids in the digestion of fats. It may also relieve symptoms of indigestion and bloating.

6. **Heart Health:** Some studies suggest that curcumin may improve heart health by improving endothelial function, reducing inflammation, and lowering the risk factors associated with heart disease.

7. **Brain Health:** Curcumin has shown promise in supporting brain health. It can increase the production of brain-derived neurotrophic factor (BDNF), a growth hormone that functions in the brain, potentially delaying or reversing brain diseases and age-related cognitive decline.

8. **Cancer Prevention:** Curcumin has demonstrated anti-cancer properties and may help prevent and treat certain types of cancer. It inhibits the growth of cancer cells and suppresses the spread of tumors.

9. **Depression and Anxiety:** Some research suggests that curcumin may have a positive impact on mood disorders like depression and anxiety. It can increase brain levels of serotonin and dopamine, neurotransmitters associated with mood regulation.

10. **Skin Health:** Turmeric is used in skincare for its anti-inflammatory and antioxidant properties. It may help reduce acne, promote wound healing, and improve overall skin appearance.

11. **Immune Support:** Turmeric's immune-boosting properties may help the body defend against infections and support overall immune function.

12. **Liver Health:** Turmeric supports liver function by aiding in the detoxification process. It may help protect the liver from damage caused by toxins and alcohol.

13. **Weight Management:** Curcumin may assist in weight management by regulating metabolism and reducing inflammation in fat tissues.

14. **Diabetes Management:** Some studies suggest that curcumin may improve insulin sensitivity and help lower blood sugar levels in individuals with type 2 diabetes.

It is important to note that while turmeric is a versatile spice with numerous health benefits, the absorption of curcumin is limited when consumed on its own. To enhance absorption, it is often recommended to consume turmeric with black pepper, which contains pipevine, a compound that improves curcumin's bioavailability.

Turmeric can be incorporated into various dishes, such as curries, soups, stews, and rice dishes. Turmeric supplements containing curcumin are also available for those looking for a more concentrated source of this beneficial compound. However, it is advisable to consult with a healthcare provider before starting any new supplement regimen, especially if you have underlying health conditions or are taking medications.

WHAT ARE THE BENEFITS OF GARLIC?

Garlic (Allium sativum) is a flavorful herb widely used in cooking and traditional medicine for its numerous health benefits. It contains various.

bioactive compounds, with allicin being one of the most well-known. Here are some of the key benefits of garlic:

1. **Antimicrobial Properties:** Garlic has natural antimicrobial properties that can help fight off bacteria, viruses, and fungi. It has been used historically to treat infections, including respiratory and digestive tract infections.

2. **Immune System Support:** Garlic may boost the immune system by enhancing the activity of immune cells and stimulating the production of antibodies. Regular consumption may help reduce the risk of common colds and other infections.

3. **Heart Health:** Garlic is associated with various heart-protective benefits. It can help lower blood pressure, reduce cholesterol levels, and improve blood circulation. These effects may contribute to a lower risk of heart disease.

4. **Antioxidant Effects:** Garlic contains antioxidants that combat harmful free radicals, reducing oxidative stress in the body. This can help protect cells and tissues from damage and contribute to overall health.

5. **Anti-Inflammatory Effects:** Garlic has anti-inflammatory properties that may help reduce chronic inflammation in the body. Chronic inflammation is linked to various chronic diseases.

6. **Blood Sugar Control:** Some studies suggest that garlic may help regulate blood sugar levels and improve insulin sensitivity, making it potentially beneficial for individuals with type 2 diabetes or at risk of developing the condition.

7. **Cancer Prevention:** Garlic has been studied for its potential anti-cancer effects. It may help reduce the risk of certain types of cancer, such as stomach and colorectal cancer.

8. **Digestive Health:** Garlic can aid digestion by promoting the production of digestive enzymes and improving gut health. It may also help alleviate digestive discomfort.

9. **Respiratory Health:** Garlic's antimicrobial and anti-inflammatory properties make it useful for respiratory health. It may help relieve symptoms of respiratory infections and reduce the severity of conditions like asthma and bronchitis.

10. **Detoxification:** Garlic supports the body's natural detoxification processes, particularly in the liver. It can help the liver eliminate toxins and harmful substances from the body.

11. **Skin Health:** Garlic's anti-inflammatory and antimicrobial properties may be beneficial for skin health. It can be used topically to treat minor skin infections and acne.

12. **Hair Health:** Some people use garlic-infused oils or garlic-based hair products to promote hair growth and reduce dandruff.

13. **Bone Health:** Garlic may have a positive impact on bone health by increasing bone density and reducing the risk of osteoporosis.

14. **Weight Management:** While not a weight loss miracle, garlic may support weight management by promoting feelings of fullness and reducing appetite.

15. **Anti-Aging:** Garlic's antioxidant properties may contribute to its anti-aging effects, helping maintain healthy skin and overall vitality.

It is worth noting that while garlic offers numerous health benefits, it can also cause bad breath and digestive discomfort in some individuals. Garlic supplements are available for those who want to avoid these side effects. As with any dietary supplement or change in diet, it is a good idea to consult with a healthcare provider, especially if you have specific health concerns or are taking medications.

Natural remedies to help with migraines.

Migraines headaches can be debilitating, and finding relief often requires a combination of strategies. While natural remedies may not eliminate migraines entirely, they can help reduce the frequency and severity of attacks and provide relief when a migraine occurs. Here are some natural remedies and lifestyle changes that may help with migraines:

1. **Stay Hydrated:** Dehydration can trigger migraines in some individuals. Ensure you are drinking enough water throughout the day to stay well-hydrated.
2. **Dietary Changes:** Identify and avoid trigger foods that can bring migraines. Common triggers include caffeine, alcohol, aged cheeses, processed meats, and artificial additives like MSG. Maintain regular meal schedules to avoid low blood sugar, which can also trigger migraines.
3. **Magnesium:** Magnesium supplements may help reduce the frequency and intensity of migraines, particularly for individuals with magnesium deficiency. Consult with a healthcare provider for the appropriate dosage.

4. **Riboflavin (Vitamin B2):** Vitamin B2 supplements (riboflavin) have shown some promise in reducing migraine frequency. A typical dose is 400 mg per day.

5. **Coenzyme Q10 (CoQ10):** CoQ10 is an antioxidant that may help reduce the frequency and severity of migraines. A typical dose is 100 mg three times a day.

6. **Butterbur:** Butterbur is an herb that has been used for migraine prevention. It should be used in a standardized form, and dosages should be determined by a healthcare provider.

7. **Lavender Oil:** Inhaling the scent of lavender oil or applying diluted lavender oil to the temples may provide relief during a migraine attack.

8. **Peppermint Oil:** Peppermint oil applied topically to the forehead and temples may help alleviate headache pain.

9. **Ginger:** Ginger has anti-inflammatory properties and may help reduce migraine symptoms. You can make ginger tea or take ginger supplements.

10. **Acupressure:** Applying pressure to specific acupressure points, like the space between the thumb and index finger, can provide relief during a migraine.

11. **Yoga and Relaxation Techniques:** Stress and tension can trigger migraines. Practices like yoga, meditation, deep breathing exercises, and progressive muscle relaxation can help reduce stress and migraine frequency.

12. **Regular Sleep Patterns:** Maintain a consistent sleep schedule by going to bed and waking up at the same time every day, even on weekends.

13. **Reduce Triggers:** Identify and avoid common migraine triggers like bright lights, loud noises, and strong odors.

14. **Adequate Sleep:** Ensure you are getting enough restful sleep. Sleep deprivation can trigger migraines.

15. **Regular Exercise:** Engage in regular physical activity, as it can help reduce the frequency and intensity of migraines. However, be cautious with intense exercise during a migraine attack.

16. **Hydrotherapy:** Applying hot or cold compresses to the head or neck may provide relief. Experiment with to see which works best for you.

It is important to note that not all remedies will work for everyone, and individual responses can vary. Keeping a migraine diary to track triggers, symptoms, and the effectiveness of different remedies can be helpful in managing migraines. Additionally, consult with a healthcare provider for personalized advice, especially if your migraines are severe, frequent, or significantly impact your daily life. They can help you develop a comprehensive migraine management plan that may include natural remedies, lifestyle changes, and medication if necessary.

What are some natural remedies for stress?

Stress is a common part of life, and managing it effectively is essential for maintaining mental and physical well-being. Here are some natural remedies and stress-relief techniques that may help reduce stress:

1. **Deep Breathing:** Practice deep breathing exercises to calm the nervous system. Try the 4-7-8 technique: inhale for a count of four, hold for seven, and exhale for eight. Repeat several times.
2. **Meditation:** Regular meditation can help reduce stress and promote relaxation. There are various meditation techniques to explore, including mindfulness meditation, guided meditation, and Transcendental Meditation.
3. **Progressive Muscle Relaxation:** Tense and then relax each muscle group in your body, starting from your toes and working your way up to your head. This technique helps release physical tension.
4. **Yoga:** Yoga combines physical postures, breathing exercises, and meditation to reduce stress and promote relaxation. Regular practice can improve flexibility, strength, and mental well-being.
5. **Exercise:** Physical activity releases endorphins, which are natural mood lifters. Engaging in regular exercise, whether it is walking, jogging, swimming, or dancing, can help reduce stress.
6. **Aromatherapy:** Certain scents, like lavender, chamomile, and rose, have calming effects. You can use essential oils in a diffuser, add them to a warm bath, or apply diluted oils to your skin.
7. **Herbal Teas:** Herbal teas like chamomile, lemon balm, and valerian root have soothing properties that can help alleviate stress and promote relaxation.

8. **Journaling:** Write down your thoughts and feelings in a journal. This can help you process emotions, gain insight into sources of stress, and identify potential solutions.

9. **Time Management:** Effective time management and organization can reduce stress related to feeling overwhelmed by tasks. Prioritize your tasks and create a schedule to stay on track.

10. **Social Support:** Spend time with friends and loved ones who provide emotional support. Talking to someone you trust about your feelings can be therapeutic.

11. **Nature and Outdoor Activities:** Spending time in nature, such as hiking, gardening, or simply taking a walk in the park, can help reduce stress and improve mood.

12. **Laughter:** Laughter triggers the release of endorphins and can help alleviate stress. Watch a funny movie, attend a comedy show, or engage in activities that make you laugh.

13. **Limit Screen Time:** Excessive screen time, especially on social media, can contribute to stress. Consider taking breaks from screens and engaging in offline activities.

14. **Mindfulness:** Practice mindfulness by staying present in the moment and observing your thoughts and feelings without judgment. Mindfulness meditation is an effective way to develop this skill.

15. **Herbal Supplements:** Certain herbs like ashwagandha, holy basil, and Rhodiola are known for their adaptogenic properties, which can help the body adapt to stress. Consult with a healthcare provider before taking herbal supplements.

16. **Massage:** A professional massage or self-massage can help relax tense muscles and reduce stress.
17. **Warm Bath:** Soaking in a warm bath with Epsom salts or aromatherapy oils can be incredibly soothing and relaxing.
18. **Art and Creativity:** Engaging in creative activities like drawing, painting, or crafting can provide an outlet for stress and promote relaxation.
19. **Limit Caffeine and Alcohol:** Excessive caffeine and alcohol intake can contribute to stress and anxiety. Reduce consumption if necessary.
20. **Sleep:** Prioritize quality sleep by maintaining a consistent sleep schedule and creating a relaxing bedtime routine.

Remember that not all remedies will work the same way for everyone, so it is essential to find what works best for you. Combining several of these natural remedies and stress management techniques can be particularly effective in reducing stress and improving overall well-being. If stress becomes overwhelming or chronic, consider seeking support from a healthcare professional or therapist to develop a personalized stress management plan.

Here are some relaxation techniques.

Relaxation techniques are strategies and practices designed to promote a state of relaxation, reduce stress, and calm the mind and body. These techniques can be valuable for managing stress, anxiety, and improving overall well-being. Here are some relaxation techniques you can try:

1. **Deep Breathing:** Deep breathing exercises can quickly induce relaxation. Try the 4-7-8 technique: Inhale deeply for a count of four, hold your breath for a count of seven, and exhale slowly for a count of eight. Repeat several times.

2. **Progressive Muscle Relaxation (PMR):** PMR involves tensing and then relaxing different muscle groups to release physical tension. Start with your toes and work your way up to your head, focusing on each muscle group.

3. **Guided Imagery:** Close your eyes and imagine a peaceful and serene place. Picture yourself there, engaging all your senses to create a vivid mental image. This can transport you to a calm and relaxing mental space.

4. **Mindfulness Meditation:** Mindfulness involves being fully present in the moment without judgment. You can practice mindfulness meditation by focusing on your breath, bodily sensations, or simply observing your thoughts as they come and go.

5. **Yoga:** Yoga combines physical postures, breathing exercises, and meditation to promote relaxation and reduce stress. There are various yoga styles to explore, from gentle and restorative to more vigorous practices.

6. **Tai Chi:** Tai Chi is a gentle form of exercise that involves slow, flowing movements and deep breathing. It promotes relaxation, balance, and mental focus.

7. **Autogenic Training:** Autogenic training involves repeating a series of self-suggestions to promote relaxation, such as "my arms are heavy and warm" or "my breathing is calm and regular."

8. **Biofeedback:** Biofeedback techniques use sensors to provide real-time information about bodily functions, such as heart rate and muscle tension. By learning to control these functions, you can reduce stress and promote relaxation.

9. **Aromatherapy:** Certain scents, like lavender, chamomile, and eucalyptus, are known for their relaxation-inducing properties. You can use essential oils in a diffuser, add them to a warm bath, or apply diluted oils to your skin.

10. **Hypnosis:** Hypnotherapy involves guided relaxation and focused attention to help individuals reach a state of deep relaxation and heightened suggestibility, which can be used for therapeutic purposes.

11. **Music and Sound Therapy:** Listening to calming music or nature sounds can help reduce stress and induce relaxation. You can also explore sound therapy practices like Tibetan singing bowl meditation.

12. **Art and Creativity:** Engaging in creative activities like drawing, coloring, or journaling can provide a relaxing outlet for self- expression and stress reduction.

13. **Breath Control Techniques:** Breathing exercises, such as diaphragmatic breathing, can help calm the nervous system and reduce stress.

14. **Warm Baths:** Soaking in a warm bath can relax tense muscles and create a sense of relaxation.

15. **Guided Relaxation Apps:** There are various mobile apps and online resources that offer guided relaxation and meditation sessions, making it easier to incorporate these practices into your daily routine.

16. **Nature and Outdoor Activities:** Spending time in nature, like hiking, gardening, or simply taking a walk in a natural setting, can be incredibly relaxing and rejuvenating.

17. **Journaling:** Writing down your thoughts and feelings in a journal can help you process emotions and relieve stress.

It is important to explore different relaxation techniques to find the ones that work best for you. Incorporating relaxation practices into your daily routine can be a valuable way to reduce stress, improve mental well-being, and enhance overall quality of life.

Benefits of meditation?

Meditation is a mind-body practice that has been used for thousands of years to promote relaxation, improve mental clarity, and enhance overall well-being. The benefits of meditation are both physical and mental, and they can have a profound impact on various aspects of your life. Here are some of the key benefits of meditation:

1. **Stress Reduction:** One of the most well-known benefits of meditation is its ability to reduce stress. Meditation triggers the relaxation response, which helps lower stress hormones like cortisol, leading to a sense of calm and relaxation.

2. **Anxiety Management:** Regular meditation practice can help reduce symptoms of anxiety disorders, including generalized anxiety disorder, social anxiety disorder, and panic disorder. It teaches individuals to manage and control anxious thoughts and feelings.

3. **Improved Emotional Well-Being:** Meditation can enhance emotional regulation, reduce symptoms of depression, and promote a more positive outlook on life. It can also increase feelings of happiness and contentment.

4. **Enhanced Concentration:** Meditation exercises the "attention muscle," improving your ability to focus and sustain attention. This heightened concentration can benefit various aspects of life, including work, study, and creative endeavors.

5. **Strengthened Self-Awareness:** Meditation encourages self-reflection and self-awareness, helping individuals gain insight into their thoughts, emotions, and behaviors. This self-awareness can lead to personal growth and positive changes.

6. **Better Sleep:** Meditation can improve the quality of sleep by relaxing the mind and body, making it easier to fall asleep and

stay asleep. It is especially beneficial for individuals with insomnia.

7. **Pain Management:** Mindfulness meditation has been shown to reduce the perception of pain and improve pain tolerance. It is often used as a complementary therapy for chronic pain conditions.

8. **Lower Blood Pressure:** Meditation can have a positive impact on blood pressure and cardiovascular health by promoting relaxation and reducing stress-related hypertension.

9. **Enhanced Resilience:** Regular meditation practice can enhance psychological resilience, helping individuals better cope with life's challenges and bounce back from adversity.

10. **Improved Relationships:** Meditation can lead to more compassionate and empathetic interactions with others. It can improve communication and reduce interpersonal conflicts.

11. **Boosted Immune System:** Some studies suggest that meditation may have immune-boosting effects, potentially enhancing the body's ability to defend against illness and infection.

12. **Spiritual Growth:** For many, meditation is a spiritual practice that fosters a deeper connection with their inner selves and a greater sense of purpose or meaning in life.

13. **Reduced Symptoms of Post-Traumatic Stress Disorder (PTSD):** Mindfulness-based meditation practices have been used in the treatment of PTSD to reduce symptoms and improve quality of life for affected individuals.

14. **Positive Brain Changes:** Brain imaging studies have shown that regular meditation can lead to structural and functional.

changes in the brain associated with memory, learning, and emotional regulation.

15. **Enhanced Creativity:** Meditation can stimulate creative thinking and problem-solving by allowing the mind to access deeper levels of consciousness and insight.

It is important to note that the benefits of meditation often become more pronounced with consistent practice over time. The type of meditation practiced, such as mindfulness meditation, loving-kindness meditation, or transcendental meditation, can also influence the specific benefits experienced. Meditation is a versatile practice, and individuals can choose the approach that best aligns with their goals and preferences.

What are some meditation apps?

There are numerous meditation apps available for both Android and iOS devices, catering to various meditation styles and preferences. Here are some popular meditation apps that you can explore:

1. **Headspace:** Headspace offers guided meditation sessions for beginners and experienced meditators alike. It covers various topics, including stress reduction, sleep improvement, and mindfulness. The app also includes "Sleep casts" for better sleep.

2. **Calm:** Calm provides guided meditation sessions, sleep stories, breathing exercises, and more. It is known for its soothing interface and calming content, making it suitable for beginners and those seeking relaxation.

3. **Insight Timer:** Insight Timer offers a vast library of free guided meditations led by meditation teachers from around the world. It includes various meditation styles, music tracks, and customizable meditation timers.

4. **Meditation & Relaxation by Breath:** Breathe (formerly known as OMG. I Can Meditate!) provides guided meditation, sleep stories, and mindfulness exercises. It offers content for reducing anxiety, improving sleep, and enhancing overall well-being.

5. **Ten percent Happier:** Created by ABC news anchor Dan Harris, 10% Happier offers meditation courses, video lessons, and interviews with meditation teachers. It is designed to make meditation more accessible and relatable.

6. **Simple Habit:** Simple Habit offers guided meditation sessions as short as 5 minutes, making it suitable for busy individuals. The app covers various topics, including stress, sleep, focus, and more.

7. **Aura:** Aura provides personalized meditation recommendations based on your mood and preferences. It offers guided sessions, sleep stories, and mindfulness exercises.

8. **The Mindfulness App:** The Mindfulness App offers guided and silent meditation sessions, as well as customizable meditation timers. It includes various mindfulness programs and reminders to practice.

9. **Smiling Mind:** Smiling Mind is designed for all ages and offers mindfulness and meditation programs tailored to different age groups, from children to adults. It is an excellent choice for families.

10. **buddhi:** buddhi is known for its meditation sessions designed for various real-life situations, such as commuting, working, and dealing with difficult emotions. It aims to integrate mindfulness into daily life.

11. **Pizizz:** Pizazz focuses on improving sleep through guided sleep stories and soundscapes. It is designed to help users fall asleep faster and wake up refreshed.

12. **MyLife Meditation (formerly Stop, Breathe & Think):** MyLife Meditation provides guided meditation sessions, emotional check-ins, and mindfulness activities tailored to your current state of mind.

13. **Omvana:** Omvana offers a wide range of guided meditations, hypnotherapy sessions, and binaural beats for meditation and relaxation.

14. **Wildflowers:** Wildflowers offers a library of guided meditation for children and teens. It is a valuable resource for teaching mindfulness and relaxation techniques to kids.

Most of these apps offer free versions with limited content and optional premium subscriptions that unlock a wider range of guided sessions and features. Explore these apps to find the one that best suits your meditation goals and preferences.

Good natural detoxifying remedies

Detoxifying the body naturally involves supporting the body's natural detoxification processes, primarily those carried out by the liver, kidneys, and lymphatic system. While there are no quick fixes or magic remedies, adopting a healthy lifestyle and incorporating certain foods and practices into your routine can help promote detoxification. Here are some natural detoxifying remedies:

1. **Stay Hydrated:** Drinking plenty of water helps flush toxins out of the body through urine and sweat. You can also add a squeeze of lemon or a few slices of cucumber to your water for extra detox benefits.

2. **Eat a Balanced Diet:** Consume a diet rich in whole foods, such as fruits, vegetables, whole grains, lean proteins, and healthy fats. Fiber from plant-based foods helps eliminate waste and toxins from the digestive system.

3. **Cruciferous Vegetables:** Foods like broccoli, cauliflower, kale, and Brussels sprouts contain compounds that support liver detoxification processes. Include these vegetables in your diet regularly.

4. **Herbal Teas:** Certain herbal teas, such as dandelion tea and milk thistle tea, can support liver health and detoxification.

5. **Green Tea:** Green tea contains antioxidants called catechins that may aid in detoxification and improve liver function.

6. **Garlic:** Garlic is known for its sulfur-containing compounds that support liver detoxification. Add fresh garlic to your meals for added flavor and detox benefits.

7. **Turmeric:** Curcumin, the active compound in turmeric, has antioxidant and anti-inflammatory properties that can support the liver and overall detoxification.
8. **Ginger:** Ginger is known for its digestive benefits and may help promote detoxification by improving digestion and reducing inflammation.
9. **Fasting or Intermittent Fasting:** Some people find benefits in intermittent fasting or periodic fasting to give the digestive system a break and promote detoxification. Consult a healthcare professional before starting any fasting regimen.
10. **Probiotics:** A healthy gut microbiome is essential for efficient detoxification. Incorporate probiotic-rich foods like yogurt, kefir, sauerkraut, and kimchi into your diet.
11. **Dry Brushing:** Dry brushing involves using a natural bristle brush to gently exfoliate the skin. It can stimulate the lymphatic system and promote detoxification through the skin.
12. **Sweating:** Regular exercise that causes you to sweat can help eliminate toxins through the skin. Activities like saunas, hot yoga, and cardio workouts can be effective.
13. **Epsom Salt Baths:** Adding Epsom salts to a warm bath can help draw out toxins from the body and promote relaxation.
14. **Reduce Exposure to Toxins:** Minimize exposure to environmental toxins by choosing natural cleaning products, reducing plastic use, and avoiding unnecessary exposure to chemicals.
15. **Hydrotherapy:** Alternating between hot and cold showers or baths can stimulate circulation and the lymphatic system.

16. **Adequate Sleep:** Quality sleep is essential for the body's natural detoxification processes. Aim for 7-9 hours of restful sleep per night.

17. **Mindful Eating:** Pay attention to your eating habits, chew food thoroughly, and eat in a calm, relaxed environment to support healthy digestion.

18. **Reduce Alcohol and Caffeine:** Limit alcohol and caffeine intake, as they can place added stress on the liver.

It is important to remember that the body's natural detoxification systems are highly efficient, and there is no need for extreme or prolonged detox diets or cleanses. Instead, focus on maintaining a balanced, healthy lifestyle that supports the body's ongoing detoxification processes. If you have specific health concerns or are considering a detoxification program, consult with a healthcare professional for personalized guidance.

What are some tips for mindful eating?

Mindful eating is a practice that involves paying full attention to the experience of eating, from the moment you select your food to the moment you take your last bite. It can help you develop a healthier relationship with food, prevent overeating, and enhance your overall well-being. Here are some tips for mindful eating:

1. **Eat Without Distractions:** Turn off the TV, put away your phone, and sit down at a designated eating space. Avoid multitasking while eating, as it can lead to mindless overeating.

2. **Engage Your Senses:** Take a moment to appreciate the appearance, aroma, and texture of your food before taking your first bite. Notice the colors, shapes, and smells.

3. **Chew Slowly and Thoroughly:** Chew your food slowly and savor each bite. This not only helps with digestion but also allows you to enjoy the flavors and textures of your meal.

4. **Put Down Your Utensils:** Between bites, put your utensils down. This encourages you to pause and assess your hunger and fullness cues.

5. **Listen to Your Body:** Pay attention to your body's hunger and fullness signals. Eat when you are hungry and stop when you are satisfied, not overly full.

6. **Check in with Your Emotions:** Before eating, take a moment to check in with your emotions. Are you eating out of hunger, boredom, stress, or habit? Identifying your emotional triggers can help you make more conscious choices.

7. **Portion Control:** Be mindful of portion sizes. Use smaller plates and serving utensils to help control portions and prevent overeating.

8. **Savor Each Bite:** As you eat, notice the taste and texture of your food. Try to identify all the ingredients in your dish.

9. **Eat with Gratitude:** Express gratitude for your food and the effort that went into preparing it. This can create a positive and mindful eating experience.

10. **Slow Down:** Eat at a leisurely pace. Put your fork down between bites and take your time to enjoy your meal.

11. **Respect Your Body:** Avoid restrictive diets and focus on nourishing your body with a balanced and varied diet. Trust your body's wisdom to guide your food choices.

12. **Practice Mindful Shopping:** When grocery shopping, make a list and stick to it. Avoid impulse purchases of unhealthy items.

13. **Mindful Cooking:** If you are preparing your meals, do so with intention and mindfulness. Engage in the cooking process and savor the experience.

14. **Accept Imperfection:** Be kind and forgiving to yourself. Mindful eating is a practice, and it is okay to have moments of mindlessness. The goal is progress, not perfection.

15. **Reflect After Eating:** After finishing your meal, take a moment to reflect on how you feel. Are you satisfied? Did you enjoy your meal? This self-awareness can help you make better choices in the future.

16. **Seek Support:** Consider joining a mindful eating group or working with a registered dietitian or therapist who specializes in mindful eating if you need additional guidance and support.

Remember that mindful eating is a skill that takes time to develop. Be patient with yourself and practice regularly. Over time, it can lead to a healthier relationship with food and a more enjoyable eating experience.

Here are some healthy meal ideas.

Healthy meal ideas can vary widely depending on your dietary preferences and restrictions, but here are some general meal ideas that can serve as a starting point for creating balanced and nutritious meals:

BREAKFAST:

1. **Oatmeal:** Top oatmeal with fresh berries, sliced bananas, and a sprinkle of nuts or seeds for added fiber and protein.

2. **Greek Yogurt Parfait:** Layer Greek yogurt with granola, honey, and mixed berries for a protein-packed breakfast.

3. **Avocado Toast:** Spread mashed avocado on whole-grain toast and top with sliced tomatoes, a poached egg, and a pinch of salt and pepper.

4. **Smoothie:** Blend spinach, frozen berries, banana, Greek yogurt, and a scoop of protein powder for a nutrient-packed smoothie.

5. **Egg Scramble:** Cook scrambled eggs with diced vegetables like bell peppers, onions, and spinach. Serve with whole-grain toast.

LUNCH:

1. **Grilled Chicken Salad:** Toss grilled chicken breast with mixed greens, cherry tomatoes, cucumber, and a vinaigrette dressing.

2. **Quinoa Bowl:** Create a quinoa bowl with roasted vegetables, chickpeas, and a tahini dressing.

3. **Vegetable Wrap:** Fill a whole grain wrap with hummus, sliced avocado, shredded carrots, cucumber, and mixed greens.

4. **Miso Soup:** Enjoy a bowl of miso soup with tofu and seaweed, served with a side of brown rice.

5. **Stir-Fry:** Stir-fry tofu or lean protein with a variety of colorful vegetables in a light stir-fry sauce. Serve over brown rice or cauliflower rice.

DINNER:

1. **Baked Salmon:** Season salmon with herbs and bake in the oven. Serve with steamed broccoli and quinoa.

2. **Vegetable Curry:** Make a vegetable curry with chickpeas, cauliflower, spinach, and a flavorful curry sauce. Serve over brown rice.

3. **Taco Salad:** Create a taco salad with lean ground turkey or tofu, black beans, lettuce, tomatoes, avocado, and a dollop of Greek yogurt as a healthier alternative to sour cream.

4. **Sweet Potato and Black Bean Bowl:** Roast sweet potatoes, black beans, and corn with spices. Top with diced avocado and a squeeze of lime.

5. **Baked Chicken and Vegetables:** Bake chicken breast with a variety of vegetables, such as carrots, bell peppers, and zucchini, seasoned with herbs and olive oil.

SNACKS:

1. **Apple Slices with Almond Butter:** Slice apples and dip them in almond butter for a satisfying and nutritious snack.

2. **Hummus and Veggie Sticks:** Enjoy raw carrot, celery, and cucumber sticks with hummus for a crunchy and healthy snack.

3. **Mixed Nuts:** A small handful of mixed nuts provides healthy fats and protein.
4. **Greek Yogurt with Berries:** Top Greek yogurt with fresh berries and a drizzle of honey for a creamy and sweet snack.
5. **Cottage Cheese with Pineapple:** Pair cottage cheese with diced pineapple for a protein-rich and slightly sweet snack.

Remember to customize these meal ideas based on your dietary preferences and any specific dietary restrictions you may have. Additionally, portion control is important to maintain a balanced diet, so be mindful of portion sizes to ensure you are getting the right amount of nutrients for your needs.

Conclusion, and tips to a healthy diet and lifestyle

Maintaining a healthy diet and lifestyle is essential for overall well-being and can significantly impact your long-term health. Here is a conclusion and some key tips to help you achieve and maintain a healthy diet and lifestyle:

CONCLUSION:

A healthy diet and lifestyle are not short-term goals but rather lifelong commitments to your well-being. Making conscious choices about

What you eat, how you move, and how you care for your physical and mental health can lead to improved energy, better mood, and reduced risk of chronic diseases. Remember that it is okay to indulge occasionally, but consistency in healthy choices is key.

TIPS FOR A HEALTHY DIET AND LIFESTYLE:

1. **Balanced Diet:** Strive for a balanced diet that includes a variety of fruits, vegetables, whole grains, lean proteins, and healthy fats. Avoid excessively processed foods, added sugars, and saturated fats.

2. **Portion Control:** Be mindful of portion sizes to avoid overeating. Use smaller plates and listen to your body's hunger and fullness cues.

3. **Stay Hydrated:** Drink plenty of water throughout the day to stay hydrated. Limit sugary drinks and excessive caffeine.

4. **Meal Planning:** Plan your meals and snacks ahead of time to make healthier choices and avoid last-minute unhealthy options.

5. **Regular Exercise:** Incorporate regular physical activity into your routine. Aim for a mix of cardiovascular exercise, strength training, and flexibility exercises.

6. **Adequate Sleep:** Prioritize quality sleep by maintaining a consistent sleep schedule and creating a relaxing bedtime routine.

7. **Stress Management:** Practice stress-reduction techniques like meditation, deep breathing, or mindfulness to manage stress effectively.

8. **Mindful Eating:** Pay attention to what and how you eat. Eat without distractions and savor each bite mindfully.

9. **Social Connections:** Maintain positive social connections and spend time with friends and loved ones. Social support is essential for mental well-being.

10. **Regular Check-ups:** Schedule regular check-ups with your healthcare provider to monitor your health and address any concerns.

11. **Limit Alcohol and Avoid Smoking:** Limit alcohol consumption and avoid smoking or using tobacco products to reduce health risks.

12. **Stay Informed:** Stay informed about nutrition, health, and wellness. Keep up with the latest research and recommendations.

13. **Set Realistic Goals:** Set achievable health and wellness goals that are specific, measurable, and time bound.

14. **Practice Self-Compassion:** Be kind to yourself and recognize that setbacks are a normal part of the journey. Celebrate your successes, no matter how small.

15. **Seek Support:** If needed, seek support from healthcare professionals, dietitians, therapists, or support groups to help you achieve and maintain your health goals.

Remember that making gradual, sustainable changes to your lifestyle is often more effective than drastic, short-term measures. Healthy habits built over time are more likely to last. Prioritize self-care and wellness and make choices that support your physical and mental health. Your health is an invaluable asset, and investing in it through a

A healthy diet and lifestyle is one of the best decisions you can make for yourself.